Academy of Nutrition and Dietetics
Pocket Guide to

Pediatric Weight Management

Second Edition

Mary Catherine Mullen, MS, RDN

Jodie Shield, MEd, RDN

Academy of Nutrition and Dietetics
Chicago, IL

eat right. Academy of Nutrition and Dietetics

Academy of Nutrition and Dietetics Pocket Guide to Pediatric Weight Management, Second Edition

ISBN 978-0-88091-996-8 (print)
ISBN 978-0-88091-997-5 (eBook)

Catalog Number 335517 (print)
Catalog Number 335517e (eBook)

10   9   8   7   6   5   4   3   2   1

For more information on the Academy of Nutrition and Dietetics, visit www.eatright.org.

Contents

List of Boxes, Tables, and Figures

Boxes

Tables

Figures

Frequently Used Abbreviations

ALT	alanine aminotransferase
AST	aspartate aminotransferase
BMI	body mass index
CDC	Centers for Disease Control and Prevention
DRI	dietary reference intake
eNCPT	electronic Nutrition Care Process Terminology
FDA	US Food and Drug Administration
HIPAA	Health Insurance Portability and Accountability Act
MNT	medical nutrition therapy
NAFLD	nonalcoholic fatty liver disease
NCP	Nutrition Care Process
NCPT	Nutrition Care Process Terminology
NHANES	National Health and Nutrition Examination Survey
NHLBI	National Heart, Lung, and Blood Institute
PA	physical activity
PAL	physical activity level
PES	problem, etiology, and signs and symptoms
PWM NPG	Pediatric Weight Management Nutrition Practice Guideline
RDN	registered dietitian nutritionist
TEE	total energy expenditure
WHO	World Health Organization

Reviewers

Emily Craft, RDN, CSP, LDN
Giant Food
Severna Park, MD

Lara Field, RDN
FEED–Forming Early Eating Decisions
Chicago, IL

Victoria Ann Hahn, MS, RDN
LAC+USC Medical Center
Los Angeles, CA

Hollie Raynor, PhD, RD
University of Tennessee, Department of Nutrition
Knoxville, TN

Linda Ro, MS, RDN, LD
Ohio Children with Medical Handicaps Program
Youngstown, OH

Christina Stella, MS, RDN, CDN, CDE
Memorial Sloan Kettering Cancer Center
New York, NY

Academy of Nutrition and Dietetics Evidence Analysis Ratings

The following ratings are used in Academy of Nutrition and Dietetics evidence analysis projects, including the Evidence-Based Pediatric Weight Management Nutrition Practice Guideline.

Strong

Definition

A **Strong** recommendation means that the work group believes that the benefits of the recommended approach clearly exceed the harms (or that the harms clearly exceed the benefits in the case of a strong negative recommendation) and that the quality of the supporting evidence is excellent/good (grade I or II). In some clearly identified circumstances, Strong recommendations may be made based on lesser evidence when high-quality evidence is impossible to obtain and the anticipated benefits strongly outweigh the harms.

Implication for Practice

Practitioners should follow a **Strong** recommendation unless a clear and compelling rationale for an alternative approach is present.

Fair

Definition

A **Fair** recommendation means that the work group believes that the benefits exceed the harms (or that the harms clearly exceed the benefits in the case of a negative recommendation), but the quality of evidence is not as strong (grade II or III). In some clearly identified circumstances, recommendations may be made based on lesser evidence when high-quality evidence is impossible to obtain and the anticipated benefits outweigh the harms.

Implication for Practice

Practitioners should generally follow a **Fair** recommendation but remain alert to new information and be sensitive to patient preferences.

Weak

Definition

A **Weak** recommendation means that the quality of evidence that exists is suspect or that well-done studies (grade I, II, or III) show little clear advantage to one approach versus another.

Implication for Practice

Practitioners should be cautious in deciding whether to follow a recommendation classified as **Weak** and should exercise judgment and be alert to emerging publications that report evidence. Patient preference should have a substantial influencing role.

Consensus

Definition

A **Consensus** recommendation means that Expert opinion (grade IV) supports the guideline recommendation even though the available scientific evidence did not present consistent results or controlled trials were lacking.

Implication for Practice

Practitioners should be flexible in deciding whether to follow a recommendation classified as **Consensus**, although they may set boundaries on alternatives. Patient preference should have a substantial influencing role.

Insufficient Evidence

Definition

An **Insufficient Evidence** recommendation means that there is both a lack of pertinent evidence (grade V) or an unclear balance between benefits and harms.

Implication for Practice

Practitioners should feel little constraint in deciding whether to follow a recommendation labeled as **Insufficient Evidence** and should exercise judgment and be alert to emerging publications that report evidence that clarifies the balance of benefit versus harm. Patient preference should have a substantial influencing role.

This section is adapted with permission from the Academy of Nutrition and Dietetics Evidence Analysis Library. https://www.andeal.org/recommendation-ratings. Accessed October 21, 2016.

Chapter 1

Pediatric Overweight and Obesity: Trends and Health Consequences

The United States is currently in the midst of an overweight/obesity crisis that affects not onl4y adults but also the nation's youth.[1,2] To accurately depict the national prevalence of childhood and adolescent overweight/obesity, it is important first to define the terms overweight and obese and then to use these definitions consistently. This chapter will provide the current overweight and obesity definitions as they apply to the pediatric population, age 2 through 18 years. It will also provide an overview of the health consequences related to pediatric overweight and obesity.

Definitions

In 2007, an Expert Committee on the Assessment, Prevention, and Treatment of Child and Adolescent Overweight and Obesity, made up of representatives from 15 health professional organizations, provided recommendations for the management of overweight and obesity in children and adolescents. The Expert Committee published a consensus document using evidence to recommend strategies for the screening, prevention, and treatment of childhood obesity.[3] The Academy of Nutrition and Dietetics Evidence-Based Pediatric Weight Management Nutrition Practice Guideline (PWM NPG) are complementary and use the Expert Committee's terminology for framing treatment recommendations.[4] The Expert Committee recommendations are discussed in greater detail in Chapters 5 and 10. The PWM NPG is discussed in Chapters 3, 4, 6, and 9. In addition, in 2010, the US Preventive

Services Task Force (USPSTF) issued revised recommendations for the screening, prevention, and treatment of childhood overweight and obesity. The USPSTF updated its terminology to be consistent with that of the Expert Committee.[5]

With regard to weight classifications, the Expert Committee recommends the following definitions[3]:

- Youth between the ages of 2 and 18 years with a body mass index (BMI) from the 85th to the 94th percentile for their age and sex should be considered *overweight*.

- Youth between the ages of 2 and 18 years with a BMI at or more than the 95th percentile for their age and sex should be considered *obese*.

- For children and adolescents with more severe obesity, an additional category (BMI greater than the 99th percentile) has been proposed to indicate a high likelihood of immediate medical problems and the urgency of intervening.

Table 1.1 summarizes pediatric weight terminology based on BMI as recommended by the Expert Committee.

Table 1.1: Terminology for Body Mass Index Categories[3,4]				
	Body Mass Index Percentile for Age and Sex			
	<5th	5th–84th	85th–94th	≥95th
Expert Committee Terminology	Underweight	Healthy weight	Overweight	Obese

In addition, more recent researchers have proposed additional definitions of severe obesity.[6] These, as well as the use of BMI *z* scores as an alternative to BMI percentiles, will be discussed more in Chapter 2 and Chapter 7.

Prevalence

Since the 1970s there has been an alarming increase in the prevalence of overweight and obesity in our nation's youth. According to the Centers for Disease Control and Prevention, childhood obesity has more than doubled in children and quadrupled in adolescents in the past 30 years.[7] Childhood obesity is a complex issue. The main causes of excess weight in youth are similar to those in adults, including individual causes such as behavior and genetics. Behaviors can include dietary patterns, physical activity, inactivity, medication use, and other exposures. Some additional contributing factors in our society include the food and physical activity environment, education and skills, and food marketing and promotion.[8]

Progress toward reducing the nation's prevalence of weight issues is monitored using data from the National Health and Nutrition Examination Survey (NHANES). The most recent NHANES data (2011 through 2014) showed that the prevalence of obesity among US youth was 17% from 2011 through 2014.[7] Overall, the prevalence of obesity was 8.9% among preschool children (2 to 5 years old), 17.5% among school-aged children (6 to 11 years old), and 20.5% among adolescents (12 to 19 years old). The same pattern was seen in both boys and girls.[9] Figure 1.1 (see page 4) presents NHANES survey data from 2011 through 2014.

From 1999 to 2000 through 2013 to 2014, a significant increase in obesity was seen; however, between 2011 and 2012 and 2013 and 2014 no changes in obesity were noted.[9]

Although the prevalence of pediatric obesity has increased nationwide, NHANES data indicate that there are significant racial/ethnic and age disparities among children and adolescents. The prevalence of obesity among non-Hispanic Asian youth (8.9%) was lower than that for non-Hispanic white (14.7%), non-Hispanic black (19.5%), and Hispanic (21.9%) youth.[9]

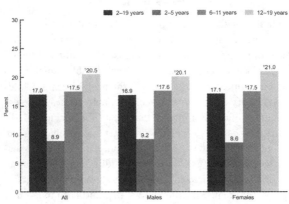

Figure 1.1: Prevalence of obesity among youth aged 2 through 19 years by sex and age: United States 2011 through 2014

Figure 1.2 compares the prevalence of obesity by race/ethnicity for adolescent boys and girls between 2 and 19 years old.[9]

The US government monitors and updates statistics on the prevalence of obesity in the pediatric population approximately every 2 years. Therefore, registered dietitian nutritionists (RDNs) and other health professionals should check the Centers for Disease Control and Prevention National Center for Health Statistics website (www.cdc.gov) for the most current pediatric obesity prevalence statistics for age, sex, and race/ethnicity.

The prevalence of childhood and adolescent obesity is also rising around the world. In 2016, The World Health Organization (WHO) put together the Commission on Ending

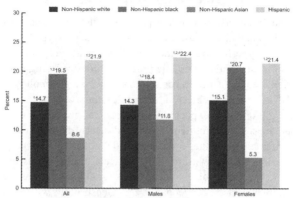

[1]Significantly different from non-Hispanic Asian persons.
[2]Significantly different from non-Hispanic white persons.
[3]Significantly different from females of the same race and Hispanic origin.
[4]Significantly different from non-Hispanic black persons.

Reprinted from National Center for Health Statistics. Prevalence of obesity among adults and youth: United States, 2011-2014. NCHS Data Brief, No. 219. www.cdc.gov /nchs/data/databriefs/db219.pdf.

Figure 1.2: Prevalence of obesity among youth aged 2 through 19 years old by sex and race/ethnicity: United States 2011 through 2014

Childhood Obesity to provide policy recommendations to governments for preventing infants, children, and adolescents from developing obesity (further discussed in Chapter 10). The WHO definitions for pediatric obesity are different from those of the Expert Committee and are based on the number of standard deviations above either the WHO growth reference median for children 5 to 19 years old or the WHO Child Growth Standards median for children under age 5. More details about the WHO definitions and current world statistics of pediatric obesity can be found in the Report of the Commission on Ending Childhood Obesity.[10]

Health Consequences

Pediatric overweight and obesity are multisystem diseases with potentially devastating consequences.[3,8-14] Type 2 diabetes, hyperlipidemia, and hypertension, as well as early maturation and orthopedic problems, are occurring with increased frequency in youth who are overweight or obese.[3,11-16] In addition, children and adolescents who are overweight or obese experience psychosocial problems, such as low self-esteem, depression, and discrimination, more commonly than other children and adolescents.[11,13,14] Finally, because children who are obese, particularly adolescents, are more likely to be overweight or obese as adults, their future health may also be in jeopardy.[12,15,16] Obese adults who were obese as children experience more rapid and serious obesity-related complications than do people who maintained a healthy weight during childhood but became obese as adults.[17] Research is now finding that the risk of pediatric overweight can begin as early as birth.[18] Box 1.1 summarizes health conditions associated with pediatric overweight/obesity.

Orthopedic Conditions

Numerous orthopedic disorders are observed more commonly in children and adolescents who are obese. Most result from the impact of increased weight on the developing skeletal system.[1,14,19]

- **Feet, leg, and hip abnormalities:** Youth who are overweight or obese can develop orthopedic abnormalities affecting the feet, legs, and hips as a result of inappropriate loading of the skeletal framework, particularly in areas involving the epiphyseal plates (unfused growth plates and softer cartilaginous bones, typically in the knee, ankle, and hip).[19] Compared with children who are not obese, children who are obese reported a greater prevalence of fractures and musculoskeletal discomfort.[19]

Box 1.1: Health Consequences of Pediatric Obesity

Orthopedic Conditions
- Slipped capital femoral epiphysis
- Blount disease

Neurologic Conditions
- Pseudotumor cerebri
- Recurrent headaches

Pulmonary Conditions
- Asthma
- Sleep disorders (eg, sleep apnea)

Gastrointestinal Conditions
- Nonalcoholic fatty liver disease
- Cholecystitis
- Gallstones
- Gastroesophageal reflux

Endocrine and Metabolic Conditions
- Type 2 diabetes
- Insulin resistance or prediabetes
- Polycystic ovary syndrome
- Hirsutism
- Excessive acne
- Acanthosis nigricans
- Early puberty
- Metabolic syndrome

Cardiovascular Diseases
- Hypertension
- Dyslipidemia
- Atherosclerosis

Psychosocial Conditions
- Low self-esteem
- Depression
- Peer rejection
- Eating disorders

- **Slipped capital femoral epiphysis:** This disorder of
  the hip's growth plate occurs between 9 and 16 years of
  age and has an incidence of approximately 11 cases per
  100,000 children.[19,20] It occurs more frequently when a
  child is overweight.[21]
- **Blount disease (*tibia vara*):** A condition that involves
  bowing of the legs and tibial torsion, Blount disease
  has been attributed to unequal or early excess weight-
  bearing. In a study conducted by Dietz and colleagues,
  approximately 80% of children with Blount disease were
  overweight or obese.[22]

Neurologic Conditions

- **Pseudotumor cerebri** is a rare neurologic disease of
  unknown origin characterized by increased pressure
  in the skull, which often causes headaches. In the past,
  pseudotumor cerebri typically occurred in middle-aged
  women, but it now occurs more frequently at an earlier
  age, particularly in youth who are overweight or obese.[23]
  Epidemiologic studies indicate a 14-fold increase in the
  prevalence of pseudotumor cerebri in patients whose
  weight is more than 10% above the ideal and a 20-fold
  increase in prevalence in people whose weight is 20%
  more than the ideal.[24]

Pulmonary Conditions

Children and adolescents who are overweight or obese often
have pulmonary complications, such as asthma and sleep
disorders.[11,12,14,16]

- **Obstructive sleep apnea** is one of the most serious problems associated with obesity and is more common among
  children who are severely obese. Obstructive sleep apnea
  is the cessation of breathing during sleep, lasting 10
  seconds or longer, and is characterized by loud snoring

and labored breathing. During these periods, oxygen levels in the blood may decrease dramatically. Studies show a strong association between pediatric obstructive sleep apnea and childhood obesity, and the condition can often result in poor school performance and disruptive behavior.[25-27]

- **Asthma:** The prevalence of obesity is reported to be significantly higher in youth with asthma than in peers without asthma.[28,29] The risk of new-onset asthma is higher among children who are overweight, and boys have an increased risk compared with girls.[29]

Gastrointestinal Conditions

Obesity is associated with several gastrointestinal problems ranging from constipation to more serious complications such as nonalcoholic fatty liver disease (NAFLD).

- **NAFLD** is a condition of growing concern because of the increasing prevalence of obesity and diabetes, which are significant risk factors. Like adults with this condition, most children with NAFLD are obese.[30] The spectrum of NAFLD ranges from isolated fatty infiltration (steatosis) to inflammation (nonalcoholic steatohepatitis, also known as NASH), fibrosis, and even cirrhosis.[30,31] The exact prevalence is hard to determine; NAFLD can occur in very young children but is more prevalent in adolescents. In addition, it is more prevalent in boys; the male to female ratio is 2 to 1. It has been reported to differ significantly by race and ethnicity: fatty liver is present in 11.8% of Hispanic children, 10.2% of Asian children, 8.6% of white children, and only 1.5% of black children.[31,32]

- **Gallstones** are more prevalent among children who are overweight and obese than among those who are healthy weight.[33]

- **Gastroesophageal reflux disease** and **constipation** are among the common pediatric gastrointestinal problems exacerbated by obesity.[34,35]

Endocrine Disorders

Impaired glucose tolerance, insulin resistance, and type 2 diabetes are some of the endocrine disorders increasingly associated with pediatric obesity.[11,14,16]

- **Type 2 diabetes:** The incidence of type 2 diabetes in children and adolescents has increased dramatically in recent years. Type 2 diabetes is widely considered a chronic, progressive disease. Among children and adolescents, it is associated with hypertension, dyslipidemia, and fatty liver disease.[36-39] In several studies, incidence of type 2 diabetes has increased from less than 5% of all new-onset pediatric diabetes diagnoses before 1994 to 30% to 50% after 1994.[37-39] Risk factors for type 2 diabetes are BMI greater than or equal to the 85th percentile; family history of diabetes; and black, Hispanic, or Native American ancestry. In addition, other risk factors include diabetes- and obesity-related conditions such as polycystic ovary syndrome (PCOS), acanthosis nigricans, or cardiovascular risk factors.[34-39]

- **Prediabetes:** Increased risk for developing type 2 diabetes, sometimes called prediabetes, is a common complication of childhood and adolescent obesity. Prediabetes is defined by moderate abnormalities in fasting plasma glucose, glucose intolerance, or hemoglobin A1c[37] and indicates a high risk for the development of diabetes.[38,39]

- **Early puberty:** Children who are obese tend to begin puberty earlier than children of healthy weight. When onset is premature, these children require an endocrinology evaluation just as children of healthy weight do.[11,14,15]

- **PCOS:** Obesity in adolescents is being increasingly linked to PCOS.[40,41] A main underlying problem is a hormonal balance. In women with PCOS, the ovaries make more androgens (male hormones that females also make) than usual.[40] Infrequent menses (fewer than nine cycles per year) is the most significant finding and should lead to further evaluation. Other findings include hirsutism, excessive acne, and acanthosis nigricans.[11]

- **Acanthosis nigricans** is a disorder that causes light-brown to black rough areas or increased skin markings, usually on the back side of the neck. It is increasingly described in children who are obese. Although it is associated with hyperinsulinemia, it is more strongly associated with a high BMI.[38,39] Up to 90% of pediatric patients with type 2 diabetes have acanthosis.[39]

Cardiovascular Disease

Youth who are obese are more likely to have risk factors for cardiovascular disease, such as high cholesterol or high blood pressure. In one study, 70% of children with obesity had at least one cardiovascular disease risk factor, and 39% had two or more.[42]

- **Hypertension** in children and adolescents seems to be increasing in both prevalence and rate of diagnosis.[33] This is due in part to the increasing prevalence of childhood obesity as well as growing awareness of this disease.[43-45] Children with obesity are three times more likely to have hypertension than children who are healthy weight. In addition, children who are overweight (particularly teens) and have elevated blood pressure may be at increased risk for hypertension as adults.[45] Childhood blood pressure and changes in BMI are consistently the most powerful predictors of adult blood pressure across all ages in both sexes.[46]

- **Dyslipidemia** is a group of disorders characterized by
  elevated levels of cholesterol, triglycerides, and low-
  density lipoproteins as well as low levels of high-density
  lipoproteins in the blood. Lipid-level abnormalities are
  among the most common obesity-related medical conditions.[47,48] More than 50% of children who are obese have
  lipid abnormalities, as measured by fasting lipid profile.
  Obesity during childhood and adolescence is associated with increased risk for major cardiovascular events
  during adulthood, independent of adult obesity status.[48]

Metabolic Syndrome

Metabolic syndrome is a clustering of risk factors for cardiovascular disease and diabetes mellitus, including increased
waist circumference, elevated blood pressure, increased triglycerides, decreased high-density lipoprotein cholesterol,
and increased blood glucose. The underlying risk factors
seem to be related to obesity and insulin resistance.[49] Currently, there is a lack of consensus on how to define metabolic
syndrome in the pediatric population. In adults, metabolic
syndrome is defined as three or more of the following risk factors: elevated waist circumference, triglyceride levels, blood
pressure, and fasting plasma glucose.[44] One study found metabolic syndrome in 4% of all children but 30% of children
who are obese.[50] Another study found that the risk of metabolic syndrome among children and adolescents who are
overweight increased by approximately 50% with each half-
unit increase in the BMI score (equivalent to an increase of
half a deviation in BMI).[49]

Psychosocial Conditions

Psychosocial issues involve psychological health and the
ability to relate to family members and peers. Childhood obesity is linked with several psychosocial problems, including
depression, low self-esteem, and eating disorders.[51,52]

- The likelihood that a child or adolescent who is severely obese will have a lower health-related quality of life was 5.5 times greater than that for a healthy child or adolescent, and similar to that for a child diagnosed with cancer.[53]

- Children and youth who were overweight and had decreased self-esteem reported increased rates of loneliness, sadness, and nervousness, and were more likely to smoke and consume alcohol.[54]

- Adolescents who are overweight are more likely to be socially isolated and peripheral to social networks than adolescents who are healthy weight.[55]

- Weight issues often cause body dissatisfaction, and researchers hypothesize that developing a negative body image places girls at risk for eating disorders.[51,56] Adolescents who are overweight or obese show higher lifetime rates of eating disorders, especially bulimia nervosa.[54] About 20% to 40% of adolescents seeking obesity interventions report symptoms of binge eating disorders.[56]

Summary

Children and adolescents who are overweight or obese face serious medical, emotional, and social consequences. As both adult and pediatric obesity remain a difficult challenge, RDNs must stay abreast of current recommendations and research pertaining to prevalence, assessment, treatment, and prevention strategies. This pocket guide blends current recommendations and evidence-based guidelines on the assessment, treatment, and prevention of pediatric obesity.

References

1. Institute of Medicine. *Accelerating Progress in Obesity Prevention: Solving the Weight of the Nation.* Washington, DC: National Academies Press; 2012.

2. US Department of Health and Human Services and US Department of Agriculture. Dietary guidelines for Americans 2015-2020. 8th ed. https://health.gov /dietaryguidelines/2015/guidelines/. Published December 2015. Accessed August 10, 2016.

3. Barlow SE. Expert Committee recommendations regarding the prevention, assessment, and treatment of child and adolescent overweight and obesity: summary report. *Pediatrics.* 2007;120(suppl 4):S164-S192.

4. Pediatric weight management (PWM) guideline (2015). Evidence Analysis Library website. www.andeal.org/topic.cfm?menu=5296&cat=5632. Accessed February 20, 2016.

5. US Preventive Services Task Force. Screening for obesity in children and adolescents: US Preventive Services Task Force Recommendation Statement. *Pediatrics.* 2010;125(2):361-367.

6. Kelly AS, Barlow SE, Rao G, et al; for the American Heart Association Atherosclerosis, Hypertension, and Obesity in the Youth Committee Council on Cardiovascular Disease in the Young, Council on Nutrition, Physical Activity and Metabolism, and Council on Clinical Cardiology. Severe obesity in children and adolescents: identification, associated health risks, and treatment approaches: a scientific statement from the American Heart Association. *Circulation.* 2013;128(15):1689-1712.

7. Childhood obesity facts. Centers for Disease Control and Prevention website. www.cdc.gov/healthyyouth /obesity/facts.htm. Updated August 27, 2016. Accessed August 15, 2016.

8. Childhood obesity causes & consequences. Centers for Disease Control and Prevention website. www.cdc .gov/obesity/childhood/causes.html. Updated June 19, 2015. Accessed August 15, 2016.

9. Ogden CL, Carroll MD, Fryar CD, Flegal KM.
    Prevalence of obesity among adults and youth: United
    States, 2011-2014. Centers for Disease Control and
    Prevention website. www.cdc.gov/nchs/data
    /databriefs/db219.pdf. Published November 2015.
    Accessed February 20, 2016.

10. Report of the Commission on ending childhood
    obesity. World Health Organization website.
    http://apps.who.int/iris/bitstream/10665/204176/1
    /9789241510066_eng.pdf?ua=. Accessed February 1,
    2016.

11. Gumani M, Birken C, Hamilton J. Childhood obesity:
    causes, consequences, and management. *Pediatr Clin
    North Am*. 2015:62(4):821-840. Accessed January 15,
    2016.

12. Biro FM, Wien M. Childhood obesity and adult
    morbidities. *Am J Clin Nutr*. 2010;91(suppl):1499S-
    1505S.

13. Barton M. Childhood obesity: a lifelong health risk.
    Acta Pharmacol Sin. 2012;33(2):189-193.

14. Han JC, Lawlor DA, Kimm SY. Childhood obesity.
    Lancet. 2010;375(9727):1737-1748.

15. Krebs NF, Himes JH, Jackson D, Nicklas TA, Guilday
    P, Styne D. Assessment of child and adolescent
    overweight and obesity. *Pediatrics*. 2007;120(suppl
    4):S193-S228.

16. Daniels SR. Complications of obesity in children and
    adolescents. *Int J Obes*. 2009;38;560-565.

17. Hoey H. Management of obesity in children differs
    from that of adults. *Proc Nutr Soc*. 2014;73(4):519-525.

18. Winter JD, Taylor Y, Mowrer L, Winter KM,
    Dulin MF. BMI at birth and overweight at age
    four. *Obes Res Clin Pract*. 2016 April 7. pii: S1871-
    403X(16)30007-2. doi: 10.1016/j.orcp.2016.03.010.
    [Epub ahead of print].

19. Taylor ED, Theim KR, Mirch MC, et al. Orthopedic complications of overweight in children and adolescents. *Pediatrics*. 2006;117(6):2167-2174.

20. Murray AW, Wilson NI. Changing incidence of slipped capital femoral epiphysis: a relationship with obesity. *J Bone Joint Surg Br*. 2008;90(1):92-94.

21. Manoff EM, Banify MB, Winell JJ. Relationship between body mass index and slipped capital femoral epiphysis. *J Pediatr Orthop*. 2005;25(6):744-746.

22. Dietz WH, Gross WL, Kirkpatrick JA. Blount disease (*tibia vara*): another skeletal disorder associated with childhood obesity. *J Pediatr*. 1982;101(5):735-737.

23. Scott HG, DeMaia EJ, Felton WL III, Nakatsuka M, Sismanis A. Increased intra-abdominal pressure and cardiac filling pressure in obesity-associated pseudotumor cerebri. *Neurology*. 1997;49(2):507-511.

24. Duncan FJ, Corbett JJ, Wall M. Incidence of pseudotumor cerebri population studies in Iowa and Louisiana. *Arch Neurol*. 1988;45(8):875-877.

25. Marcus CL, Brooks LJ, Draper KA, et al. Diagnosis and management of childhood obstructive sleep apnea syndrome. *Pediatrics*. 2012;150(3):577-584.

26. Narang I, Mathew JL. Childhood obesity and obstructive sleep apnea. *J Nutr Metab*. 2012;2012: 134202. www.ncbi.nlm.nih.gov/pmc/articles /PMC3432382/. Accessed August 15, 2016.

27. What causes aleep apnea? National Heart, Lung, and Blood Institute website. www.nhlbi.nih.gov/health /health-topics/topics/sleepapnea/causes. Updated July 10, 2012. Accessed August 15, 2016.

28. Sutherland ER. Obesity and asthma. *Immunol Allergy Clin North Am*. 2008;28(3):589-602.

29. Gilland FD, Berhane K, Islam T, et al. Obesity and the risk of newly diagnosed asthma in school-age children. *Am J Epidemiol*. 2003;158(5):406-415.

30. Bozic MA, Subbarao G, Molleston JP. Pediatric nonalcoholic fatty liver disease. *Nutr Clin Pract.* 2013;28(4):448-458.

31. Giorgio V, Prono F, Granziano F, Nobilli V. Pediatric non alcoholic fatty liver disease: old and new concepts on development, progression, metabolic insight and potential targets. *BMC Pediatr.* 2013;25(13). doi:10.1186/1471-2431-13-40

32. Chalasani N, Younossi Z, Lavine JE, et al. The diagnosis and management of non-alcoholic fatty liver disease: practice guideline by the American Association for the Study of Liver Diseases, American College of Gastroenterology, and the American Gastroenterologist Association. *Hepatology.* 2012;55(6):2005-2023.

33. Kaechele V, Wabitsch M, Thiere D, et al. Prevalence of gall bladder stone disease in obese children and adolescents: influence of the degree of obesity, sex, and pubertal development. *J Pediatr Gastroenterol Nutr.* 2006;24(1):66-70.

34. Fishman L, Lenders C, Fortunate C, Noonan C, Nurko S. Increased prevalence of constipation and fecal soiling in a population of obese children. *J Pediatr.* 2004;145:253-254.

35. Hampel H, Abraham NS, El-Serag HB. Meta-analysis: obesity and the risk for gastrointestinal reflux disease and its complications. *Ann Intern Med.* 2005;143(3):192-211.

36. Springer SC, Silverstein J, Copeland K, et al. Management of type 2 diabetes mellitus in children and adolescents. *Pediatrics.* 2013:131(2):e648-e684. http://pediatrics.aappublications.org/content/pediatrics /131/2/e648.full.pdf. Accessed August 15, 2016.

37. American Diabetes Association. Classification and diagnosis of diabetes. In: Standards of Medical of Medical Care in Diabetes—2015. *Diabetes Care.* 2015:38(suppl 1):S8-S16.

38. Copeland KC, Becker D, Gottschalk M, Hale D. Type 2 diabetes in children and adolescents: risk factors, diagnosis, and treatment. *Clin Diabetes.* 2005;23(4):181-185.

39. National diabetes fact sheet, 2011. Centers for Disease Control and Prevention website. www.cdc.gov /diabetes/pubs/pdf/ndfs_2011.pdf. Accessed November 27, 2016.

40. Polycystic ovary syndrome fact sheet. Office on Women's Health, US Department of Health and Human Services website. http://womenshealth.gov /publications/our-publications/fact-sheet/polycystic -ovary-syndrome.html#c. Updated June 8, 2016. Accessed August 20, 2016.

41. Rosenfield R. Polycystic ovary syndrome in adolescence associated with obesity. *AAP News.* 2007;28(4):20.

42. Freedman DS, Mei Z, Srinivasan R, Berenson GS, Dietz WH. Cardiovascular risk factors and excess adiposity among overweight children and adolescents: the Bogalusa Heart Study. *J Pediatr.* 2007;150(1):12-17.e2.

43. May AL, Kuklina EV, Yoon PW. Prevalence of cardiovascular disease risk factors among US adolescents, 1999–2008. *Pediatrics.* 2012:129(6):1035-1041.

44. Expert panel on integrated guidelines for cardiovascular health and risk reduction in children and adolescents: summary report. National Heart, Lung, and Blood Institute website. www.nhlbi.nih .gov/files/docs/guidelines/peds_guidelines_full.pdf. Published October 2012. Accessed May 12, 2017.

45. Parker ED, Sinaiko AR, Kharbanda EO, et al. Change in weight status and development of hypertension. *Pediatrics.* 2016;137(3):1-9.

46. Luma GB, Spiotta RT. Hypertension in children and adolescents. *Am Fam Physician.* 2006;73(9):1558-1568. www.aafp.org/afp/20060501/1558.html. Accessed March 24, 2009.

47. Kavey RE, Daniels SR, Lauer RM, Atkins DL, Hayman LL, Taubert K. American Heart Association guidelines for primary prevention of atherosclerotic cardiovascular disease beginning in childhood. *Circulation.* 2003;107(4):1562-1566.

48. Daniels SR, Greer FR, Committee on Nutrition. Lipid and cardiovascular health in childhood. *Pediatrics.* 2008;122(1):198-208.

49. Cook S, Weitzman M, Aunger P, Nguyen M, Dietz W. Prevalence of metabolic syndrome phenotype in children and adolescents: findings from the third National Health and Nutrition Examination Survey, 1988-1994. *Arch Pediatr Adolesc Med.* 2003;157(8):821-827.

50. Weiss R, Dziura J, Burgert TS, et al. Obesity and the metabolic syndrome in children and adolescents. *N Engl J Med.* 2004;350(23):2362-2374.

51. Morrison KM, Shin S, Tarnopolsky M, Taylor VH. Association of depression and health related quality of life with body composition and youth with obesity. *J Affect Disord.* 2015;172:18-23.

52. Halfon N, Larson K. Slusser W. Associations between obesity and comorbid mental health, developmental, and physical health conditions in a nationally representative sample of US children aged 10 to 17. *Acad Pediatr.* 2013(1):13:6-13.

53. Schwimmer JB, Burwinkle TM, Varni JW. Health-related quality of life of severely obese children and adolescents. *JAMA.* 2003;289(14):1813-1819.

54. Strauss RS. Childhood obesity and self-esteem. *Pediatrics*. 2000;105(1):1-5.

55. Strauss RS, Pollack HA. Social marginalization of overweight children. *Arch Pediatr Adolesc Med*. 2003;157(8):746-752.

56. Latz Y, Stein D. A review of the psychological and familial perspectives of childhood obesity. *J Eat Disord*. 2013;1:7. doi: 10.1186/2050-2974-1-7.

Chapter 2

Identification of Overweight and Obesity and Obesity Risk Assessment

This chapter provides an overview of the current recommendations on the identification and universal screening of overweight and obesity risk in children and adolescents. In addition, this chapter will discuss recommendations for the assessment of children or adolescents identified as obese or overweight with obesity-related health risks.

To prevent and treat obesity in children and adolescents, health professionals must correctly identify those who are overweight or obese. Health professionals should use body mass index (BMI) to diligently screen all adolescents and children older than 2 years for overweight or obesity and conduct further assessments as needed. In addition, they should become familiar with risk factors for childhood and adolescent obesity to initiate management and prevention strategies as early as possible.[1-3] According to the World Health Organization (WHO) growth charts, children under the age of 2 years with a weight for length that is higher than the 98th percentile are classified as having a high weight for length.[4]

Screening for Obesity

Body Mass Index

As discussed in Chapter 1, experts in the field have chosen to use BMI to define obesity and overweight in children and adolescents over the age of 2 years. Interpretation of BMI depends on the child's age and sex. Age is important because as children grow, their body fatness changes. Additionally, body fatness differs as girls and boys mature. Therefore, BMI is plotted according to sex-specific charts published by the Centers for Disease Control and Prevention (CDC).[5] Box 2.1 lists several other factors to consider when using BMI to screen for obesity or overweight.[3,5-7]

Box 2.1: Considerations When Using Body Mass Index to Screen for Obesity[3-6]

- Body mass index (BMI) is an effective screening tool, but it is not a diagnostic tool. It is important to assess a child or adolescent for health concerns and risk factors beyond weight.

- BMI growth curves allow health professionals to track BMI throughout childhood and adolescence. It is important to focus on the change in growth patterns or percentiles over time and address concerns before the child reaches the 95th percentile.

- BMI charts should only be used for children older than 2 years. For children younger than 2 years, the World Health Organization weight-for-length growth charts should be used to evaluate their weight in relationship to their length/stature.

- A high BMI can be an indicator of high body fatness. BMI does not measure body fat directly, but research has shown that BMI is correlated with more direct measures of body fat.

- Pubertal status influences measures of weight relative to stature, such as BMI. For early- or late-maturing children, these indexes should be interpreted with caution.

- Some children and adolescents may have a high BMI for their age and sex because of a large lean body mass from physical activity, high muscularity, or frame size.

- In the United States, BMIs for age and sex usually decrease and reach a minimum at approximately 4 or 5 years of age before beginning a gradual increase through adolescence and most of adulthood. This upward trend through adolescence has been termed adiposity rebound (AR). Rapid growth in body fat characterizes this phase of development and includes an increase in both fat cell size (hypertrophy) and number (hyperplasia). Numerous studies have reported that an early AR, occurring before age 4 to 6 years, is associated with an increased risk of overweight in adolescence and adulthood.

To evaluate BMI, clinicians use percentile cutoffs to compare values for a given child with values for healthy children of the same age and sex from a national sample.[5] As discussed in Chapter 1, the Expert Committee on the Assessment, Prevention, and Treatment of Child and Adolescent Overweight and Obesity recommendeds using the following percentile cutoffs for children aged 2 to 20 years[1]:

- **Overweight:** BMI between the 85th and the 94th percentiles for age and sex
- **Obese:** BMI greater than or equal to the 95th percentile for age and sex
- **Severe obesity with increased medical risks:** BMI greater than the 99th percentile for age and sex

In 2013, the American Heart Association Atherosclerosis, Hypertension and Obesity in Youth Committee recommended defining severe obesity in children age 2 years or older and in adolescents as having a BMI greater than or equal to 120% of the 95th percentile or absolute BMI greater than or equal to 35, whichever is lower based on age and sex.[8]

The Expert Committee recommends that physicians and allied health care providers assess the weight status of all children and adolescents at least yearly. This assessment includes calculating height, weight, and BMI and plotting those measures on standard growth charts. The following four steps should be taken to ensure accurate tracking of BMI.[1,5,8]

1. Accurately measure height and weight (see Appendix C, page 135).
2. Calculate BMI using one of the methods in Box 2.2. (see page 24)
3. Plot BMI on the appropriate CDC BMI-for-age-and-sex growth chart. These charts can be accessed and downloaded from the CDC website (http://cdc.gov /growthcharts).
4. Record BMI and BMI percentile in the patient's chart.

Box 2.2: Methods for Calculating Body Mass Index[1]

Mathematical formulas

- Body mass index (BMI) = [Weight (kg)/Height squared (cm²)] × 10,000
- BMI = [Weight (lb)/Height squared (in²)] × 703

Tools

- Online BMI calculator (https://nccd.cdc.gov/dnpabmi/Calculator.aspx)

Most facilities now use electronic medical records in which percentiles are calculated and growth charts are plotted electronically. These applications provide an exact percentile (eg, 96th percentile).[9]

BMI z scores

The BMI z score, an alternative to BMI percentile, is now widely used in research and clinical studies in youth. In addition, many practitioners have started to use it in clinical practice. The BMI z score is defined as the BMI of a child or adolescent transformed into the number of standard deviations above or below the study population mean. BMI z scores, like percentiles, allow comparison of weight change across different ages and sexes but are more sensitive to quantified changes in weight status.[10] Some electronic medical record programs automatically generate BMI z scores.

The nutrition anthropometry software program NutStat, contained within the Epi Info program, calculates percentiles and z scores for each measurement testing the CDC reference data. It is available to download at no charge from the CDC website.[9,11] The Academy of Nutrition and Dietetics NutriCare Tools app helps calculate BMI, BMI percentiles, and z scores.

Waist Circumference

Although waist circumference provides a better estimate of abdominal fat than BMI,[11] the Expert Committee does not recommend its use to evaluate pediatric weight because specific guidance and data are insufficient.[1]

Triceps Skinfold Thickness

The Expert Committee recommends against the routine clinical use of triceps skinfold thickness measurements to assess obesity in children because they are difficult to measure accurately without careful training and experience. In addition, reference data are not readily available for children.[1]

Identification of Additional Risk Factors for Obesity

In addition to using BMI, health professionals should assess children and adolescents for risk factors and characteristics associated with childhood overweight and obesity. Identification of potential risk factors and characteristics associated with a high BMI can decrease future health problems if treatment or prevention strategies are started early. Potential contributing factors include the following[1-3,12]:

- Having one or both parents overweight.
- Living in families with low incomes.
- Having chronic illness or disabilities that limit mobility.
- Being a member of certain racial/ethnic groups, such as preadolescent and adolescent African American girls, Hispanics, Native Americans, or Alaska Natives. (Refer to Chapter 1 for more information about prevalence data for different racial/ethnic groups.)

In addition, many lifestyle factors related to diet and nutrient intake and physical activity/sedentary behaviors may also be linked with a greater likelihood of increased BMI.[1,3,8,13] According to the Expert Committee, health care providers should qualitatively assess the dietary patterns and levels of physical activity and sedentary behaviors of all pediatric patients at each well-child visit or more frequently if the patient is overweight or obese.[1] The purpose of this assessment is to identify risks and provide anticipatory guidance accordingly (see Boxes 2.3 and 2.4). Nutrition risk screening tools should be used for well-child visits.[14] Chapter 10 provides a more detailed discussion along with current evidence-based research for diet and physical activity behaviors associated with childhood overweight and obesity.

Screening for Health Risks Associated with Obesity

The Expert Committee has established recommendations for assessing obesity-related risk factors in children and adolescents (see Box 2.5).[1]

Box 2.3: Qualitative Assessment of Dietary Patterns[1]

The Expert Committee recommends that qualitative assessment of dietary patterns should be done for all pediatric patients at a minimum at each well-child visit. The assessment should include the identification of the following dietary practices:

- Frequency of eating outside the home at fast-food establishments or restaurants
- Excessive consumption of sweetened beverages
- Consumption of excessive portion sizes for age

Additional factors to consider include the following:

- Excessive consumption of 100% fruit juice
- Breakfast consumption (frequency and quality)
- Excessive consumption of energy-dense foods
- Low consumption of fruits and vegetables
- Meal frequency and snacking patterns (including quality)
- Self-efficacy and readiness to change of patient or family

Box 2.4: Qualitative Assessment of Physical Activity and Sedentary Behaviors[1]

The Expert Committee recommends that assessment of physical activity and sedentary behaviors should be done for all pediatric patients at a minimum at each well-child visit. The assessment should include the following general areas:

- Whether the child is meeting recommendations of 60 minutes of at least moderate physical activity each day

- Barriers to physical activity

- Levels of sedentary behaviors (including daily hours of watching television, playing video games, and using the computer)

- Environment and social support

- Family or patient's self-efficacy and readiness to change

Box 2.5: Universal Assessment for Obesity-Related Health Risks[1]

Calculate and plot body mass index (BMI) at all well-child visits. BMI should serve as a starting point for classifying health risks.

- Children or adolescents with a BMI between the 5th and 84th percentiles have lower obesity-related health risks, but they should still be assessed for other risk factors, such as parental obesity, family medical history, and current diet and physical activity behaviors. These children and their families should receive preventive counseling that focuses on targeted behaviors and identified risks.

- Children and adolescents with a BMI between the 84th and 94th percentiles (overweight) have an increased likelihood of obesity-related health risks due to the influences of parental obesity, family medical history, current lifestyle habits, cardiovascular risks, and BMI trajectory. Preventive counseling should be given unless health risks are identified and treatment intervention is indicated.

- Children or adolescents with a BMI more than the 95th percentile (obese) are very likely to have obesity-related health risks and should be directed to intervention.

Assessment

If a child or adolescent has a positive screen for obesity or overweight with evidence of health risks, an overall assessment should be completed. Box 2.6 lists the recommended components of an assessment.[1,3] At the end of the overall assessment, health care providers will be able to help the patient and caregivers determine the most appropriate treatments for the child or adolescent,[1,2] including referral to a registered dietitian nutritionist for a nutrition assessment (see Chapter 4), nutrition intervention (see Chapter 6), and nutrition monitoring and evaluation (see Chapter 9).

Box 2.6: Components of an Overweight- or Obesity-Related Health Assessment

- Medical history
- Family history
- Review of symptoms
- Dietary and physical activity assessment
- Evaluation of patient or family's readiness to change behavior
- Clinical data:
  - Physical examination
  - Laboratory test values

Medical History

A thorough medical history provides information to identify any obesity-related risk for future disease and diagnose any underlying syndromes to identify any health complications related to obesity.[1,3,8]

Family History

Physicians and allied health care providers should obtain a focused family history to assess the risks of current or future comorbidities associated with a child or adolescent's overweight or obese status. The following conditions are recommended for evaluation (coming from first- or second-degree relatives)[1,3,8]:

- Obesity
- Type 2 diabetes mellitus
- Cardiovascular disease (particularly hypertension and dyslipidemia)
- Early death resulting from heart disease or stroke

Review of Systems

Health complications—which range from chronic complications of mild hypertension, dyslipidemia, and insulin resistance to acute complications, such as pseudotumor cerebri, sleep apnea, obesity hypoventilation, and orthopedic problems—influence the intensity of treatment.[1,3, 15] (See Chapter 1 for information concerning health complications associated with pediatric obesity.) Box 2.7 (see page 30) provides a list of symptoms associated with obesity-related health conditions that a health care provider might identify when completing a medical history for an obese or overweight child or adolescent.[1,3]

Dietary and Physical Activity Assessment

As previously discussed, dietary and physical activity and sedentary behaviors should be qualitatively assessed at each well-child visit.[1] If a child or adolescent is identified as obese or as overweight with health risks, a more detailed dietary (nutrition) and physical activity assessment should be completed to determine the most appropriate treatment (see Chapter 4).

Readiness to Change

Evaluation of the patient and parents' psychological readiness to change is an important first step in effective weight-control counseling. Attempting to initiate a weight-management

Box 2.7: Symptoms Associated with Obesity-Related Health Conditions

- Sleep apnea or snoring
- Shorter sleep time or restlessness
- Shortness of breath
- Wheezing
- Recurrent abdominal pain
- Heartburn or epigastric pain
- Frequent headaches
- Polyuria or polydipsia
- Amenorrhea or oligomenorrhea (irregular menses [< 9 cycles per year])
- Hip or knee pain
- Depression
- Problems with social interaction
- Anxiety, school avoidance, social isolation
- Poor self-esteem
- Body dissatisfaction
- History of eating disorders (binge eating, bulimia)

program for children, adolescents, or families who are not ready to change may be detrimental because of the potentially negative impact on self-esteem and impairment of further weight loss.[1,3,8]

Unless a serious complication of obesity exists, give families who are not ready to change information about the health consequences of obesity and let them know help is available when they are ready. Health professionals should continue to foster a positive relationship with these patients and their families so that treatment may be possible in the future.[1,3] Refer to Chapter 8 for more information about behavior change.

Physical Examination Data

Each child who is overweight or obese should have a complete physical examination.[1,3] This examination may be initiated as part of a well-child visit, during the screening for overweight or obesity.

Growth Assessment

An important component of the physical examination is an evaluation of growth.[1,3,14] Height for age, weight for age, and BMI should be plotted on growth charts. Weight velocity and height velocity should also be used to evaluate growth. Determine weight change or height change velocity by plotting previous weights and heights on the CDC growth curve or, if available already, electronically recording the values in the medical record. Weight velocity can be used to assess the risk of childhood obesity. The child's weight is accelerating if the charted weight is trending upward and crossing two percentile lines, and this situation warrants further assessment or a determination of childhood obesity (see Chapter 4). Children younger than 2 years who have a growth trend that crosses two percentile lines on the length-for-weight chart have the highest prevalence of obesity 5 to 10 years later.[8,14,16]

Puberty is a time for major increases in weight and height, so adequate nutrition is needed. Therefore, pubertal status should be determined for adolescents before a treatment plan is developed. Sexual maturation is a very useful way to assess the stage of puberty and corresponding nutrition needs.[8,9] Development of secondary sexual characteristics can be evaluated using sexual maturity ratings, often called Tanner staging (see Table 2.1, page 32).[9,17] Girls experience their most rapid growth in height (3 to 5 inches) between stages 2 and 3. Boys experience their most rapid growth in height between stages 3 and 4. Alterations in body composition, changes in quantity and distribution of fat, and enlargement of many organs characterize this growth spurt.[8,9]

Table 2.1: Tanner Stages of Pubertal Development		
Stage	Boys	Girls
1	Prepubertal	Prepubertal
2	Enlargement of scrotum and testes, reddening of scrotal skin Sparse growth of slightly pigmented hair at base of penis Decrease in total body fat	Breast budding with areolar enlargement Sparse growth of slightly pigmented hair along labia Accelerated growth
3	Further growth of the testes and scrotum, enlargement of penis (increased length) Darker, coarser, curlier, more dispersed pubic hair Increased muscle mass Voice begins to break	Further enlargement of breasts and areola Pubic hair is darker, coarser, curlier, more dispersed Peak linear growth velocity Axillary hair Acne
4	Still further growth of genitalia Adult-type hair but not extending to thighs Peak linear growth velocity Voice change Axillary hair	Projection of the areola and papilla to form a secondary mound Adult-type hair but not extending to thighs Linear growth deceleration Menarche[a]
5	Adult genitalia Adult pubic hair extending to thighs Linear growth slows and ceases Muscle mass continues to increase Facial hair present	Adult breast with projection of papilla only Adult pubic hair extending to thighs Linear growth slows and ceases

[a] Girls typically experience most linear growth before the onset of menarche. They grow an average of only 2 inches after menarche. However, girls who enter puberty at an earlier age may experience more linear growth after menarche.

Adapted with permission from the Academy of Nutrition and Dietetics. See reference 9.

A child with less than expected height compared with average parental height or expected linear growth should be evaluated for endocrine or congenital conditions. Children with certain genetic or hormonal syndromes may have short stature, usually at or less than the fifth percentile of height for age. Other possible characteristics include a family history of obesity, mental impairment, and delayed bone growth.[3,15]

Other Components

In addition to a growth evaluation, the Expert Committee recommends that a thorough physical examination be conducted that includes the following measurements[1]:

- **Pulse:** Measured in the standard pediatric manner.
- **Signs associated with comorbidities of overweight and obesity:** Give careful attention to the health conditions associated with childhood obesity (see Chapter 1). *Specific findings will lead to additional diagnostic testing and consultation with pediatric subspecialists. For example, if acanthosis nigricans is observed, a fasting blood glucose test is indicated and referral to a pediatric endocrinologist may be needed.*[1,3]
- **Blood pressure:** As discussed in Chapter 1, hypertension is more prevalent among children who are overweight or obese than those who are healthy weight. Although the cause of hypertension is not clear, there is often an immediate reduction in blood pressure after weight loss.[1,18, 19] See Box 2.8 (see page 34) for guidelines for evaluating blood pressure in children and adolescents who are obese.[20]

Laboratory Test Data

Recommended laboratory tests will be determined by the degree of overweight or obesity, family history, and results of the physical exam. See Table 2.2 (see page 34) for the Expert Committee's recommendations for laboratory assessment of medical risks of childhood obesity.[1,3]

Box 2.8: Evaluation of Blood Pressure in Children and Adolescents Who Are Obese[2,3,12,19]

- Use of an appropriate size blood pressure cuff is essential. The bladder of the cuff must be large enough to cover 80% of the arm. Using a cuff that is too small may yield falsely elevated readings.

- Use blood pressure tables developed by the National High Blood Pressure Education Program based on sex, age, and height to interpret and track blood pressure management.

- Keep in mind that in children and adolescents, three or more readings more than the 95th percentile for either systolic or diastolic blood pressure indicate hypertension.

Table 2.2: Laboratory Assessment of Medical Risks Associated with Childhood Obesity[1,3]

BMI[a] Percentile for Age and Sex	Risk Factors	Recommended Laboratory Tests
85th–94th	None	Fasting lipid profile
85th–94th	If patient is age 10 years or older and has other risk factors, test biannually.	Fasting lipid profile AST[b] ALT[c] Fasting plasma glucose
≥95th	Conduct tests starting at age 10 years, even in absence of risk factors. Repeat biannually.	Fasting lipids AST ALT Fasting plasma glucose

[a] BMI = body mass index.

[b] AST = aspartate aminotransferase

[c] ALT = alanine aminotransferase

Lipid Levels

Blood lipids outside the clinical range of normal are frequently present with children and adolescents who are overweight or obese.[12,15] Therefore, screening is recommended for all children and adolescents who are overweight or obese. The National Heart, Lung, and Blood Institute (NHLBI) has published acceptable, borderline, and high or low concentrations for lipids and lipoproteins for children and adolescents, which are in accordance with the National Education Program Expert Panel on Blood Cholesterol Levels in Children and are shown in Table 2.3 (see page 36).[12]

Screening for Type 2 Diabetes

The incidence of type 2 diabetes in children is increasing, and most children with type 2 diabetes are overweight or obese.[14,21,22] Diagnosis of children with type 2 diabetes typically occurs in children older than 10 years and in mid to late puberty. As the childhood population becomes increasingly obese, type 2 diabetes may be expected to occur in younger children.[1,21,22] See Box 2.9 (page 37) for current screening recommendations.[21,22]

Other Laboratory Data

Depending on the findings from the physical examination and history, other possible laboratory tests include the following[1,3]:

- Liver enzymes: Elevated liver enzymes can be associated with fatty liver, fatty fibrosis, or cirrhosis.
- Thyroid function test: If a child or adolescent has short stature, a thyroid function test and a hand-wrist radiograph for bone age may be warranted.
- Morning serum cortisol level and 24-hour urinary cortisol secretion: These tests will be diagnostic if Cushing syndrome is considered.

Table 2.3: Acceptable, Borderline-High, and High Plasma Lipid, Lipoprotein, and Apolipoprotein Concentrations (mg/dL) for Children and Adolescents[12a]

Category	Acceptable	Borderline	High
Total cholesterol	<170	170–199	≥200
Low-density lipoprotein cholesterol	<110	110–29	≥130
Non–high-density lipoprotein cholesterol	<120	120–144	≥145
Apolipoprotein B	<90	90–109	≥110
Triglyceride			
0–9 years	<75	75–99	≥100
10–19 years	<120	90–129	≥130

Category	Acceptable	Borderline	Low[b]
High-density lipoprotein cholesterol apolipoprotein A-1	>45	40–45	<40
	>120	115–120	<115

[a] Values for plasma lipid and lipoprotein levels are from the National Cholesterol Education Program (NCEP) Expert Panel on Cholesterol Levels in Children, Non–HDL-C values from the Bogalusa Heart Study are equivalent to the NCEP Pediatric Panel cutoff points for LDL-C values for plasma Apolipoprotein B and Apolipoprotein A-1 are from the national health and Nutrition Examination Survey.

[b] The cutoff points for high and borderline high represent approximately the 95th and 75th percentiles, respectively. Low cutoff points for HDL-C and Apolipoprotein A-1 represent approximately 100th percentile.

Box 2.9: Testing for Type 2 Diabetes in Children[a]

Criteria

Test children who are overweight (body mass index > 85th percentile for age and sex, weight for height > 85th percentile, or weight > 120% of ideal body weight) and who have any two of the following risk factors:

- Family history of type 2 diabetes in a first- or second-degree relative
- Race/ethnicity (Native American, African American, Latino, Asian, or Pacific Islander)
- Signs of insulin resistance or conditions associated with insulin resistance (acanthosis nigricans, hypertension, dyslipidemia, polycystic ovary syndrome) or a birth weight that is small for gestational age
- Maternal history of diabetes or gestational diabetes mellitus during the child's gestation

Age of initiation

Age 10 years or at onset of puberty if puberty occurs at a younger age

Frequency

Every 3 years

---

[a] Clinical judgment should be used to test for diabetes in high-risk patients who do not meet these criteria.

Adapted with permission from the American Diabetes Association. See reference 22.

Other Medical Tests and Procedures

Depending on physical findings, additional diagnostic tests may be ordered to confirm a medical diagnosis. These tests and procedures may include, but are not limited to, the following[1,3,8]:

- Endoscopy
- Liver biopsy
- Magnetic resonance imaging of the liver
- Polysomnography
- Sleep studies

References

1. Barlow SE. Expert Committee recommendations regarding the prevention, assessment, and treatment of child and adolescent overweight and obesity. *Pediatrics.* 2007;120(suppl 4):S164-S192.

2. Institute of Medicine. *Accelerating Progress in Obesity Prevention: Solving the Weight of the Nation.* Washington, DC: National Academies Press; 2012.

3. Krebs NF, Himes JH, Jackson D, Nicklas TA, Guilday P, Styne D. Assessment of child and adolescent overweight and obesity: summary report. *Pediatrics.* 2007;120(suppl 4):S193-S228.

4. Growth chart training: using the WHO growth Charts. centers for Disease Control and Prevention website. www.cdc.gov/nccdphp/dnpao/growthcharts/who/using/assessing_growth.htm. Accessed August 20, 2016.

5. About child and teen BMI. Centers for Disease Control and Prevention website. www.cdc.gov/healthyweight/assessing/bmi/childrens_bmi/about_childrens_bmi.html. Accessed August 15, 2016.

6. 2000 CDC growth charts for the United States: methods and development. Centers for Disease Control and Prevention website. www.cdc.gov/growthcharts/cdc_charts.htm. Accessed January 8, 2017.

7. National Health and Nutrition Examination Survey (NHANES): laboratory procedures manual. Centers for Disease Control and Prevention website. www.cdc.gov/nchs/data/nhanes/nhanes_11_12/2011-12_laboratory_procedures_manual.pdf. Accessed August 20, 2016.

8. Academy of Nutrition and Dietetics. Weight Management. Pediatric Nutrition Care Manual website. www.nutritioncaremanual.org/topic. cfm?ncm_category_id=13&lvl=144636&ncm_ toc_id=144636&ncm_heading=Nutrition%20Care. Accessed March 15, 2016.

9. Leonberg BL. *Academy of Nutrition and Dietetics Pocket Guide to Pediatric Nutrition Assessment.* 2nd ed. Chicago, IL: Academy of Nutrition and Dietetics; 2013.

10. Academy of Nutrition and Dietetics. Position of the Academy of Nutrition and Dietetics: interventions for the prevention and treatment of pediatric overweight and obesity. *J Acad Nutr Diet.* 2013;113(10):1375-1394.

11. A SAS program for the 2000 CDC growth charts (ages 0 to <20 years). Centers for Disease Control and Prevention website. www.cdc.gov/nccdphp/dnpao /growthcharts/resources/sas.htm. Accessed March 10, 2016.

12. Kelly AS, Barlow SE, Rao G, Ing TH, Hayman LL, Steinberger J, et al; for the American Heart Association Atherosclerosis, Hypertension, and Obesity in the Youth Committee Council on Cardiovascular Disease in the Young, Council on Nutrition, Physical Activity and Metabolism, and Council on Clinical Cardiology. Severe obesity in children and adolescents: identification, associated health risks, and treatment approaches: a scientific statement from the American Heart Association. *Circulation.* 2013;128(15):1689-1712

13. Pediatric Weight Management (PWM) Guideline (2015). Evidence Analysis Library website. www.andeal.org/topic.cfm?menu=5296&cat=5632. Accessed February 20, 2016.

14. Holt K, Wooldridge N, Story M, Sofka D, eds. *Bright Futures: Nutrition.* 3rd ed. Elk Grove Village, IL: American Academy of Pediatrics; 2011. https://brightfutures.aap.org/materials-and-tools/nutrition-and-pocket-guide/Pages/default.aspx. Accessed March 1, 2016.

15. Gumani M, Birken C, Hamilton J. Childhood obesity: causes, consequences, and management. *Pediatr Clin North Am.* 2015:62(4):821-840.

16. Taveras EM, Rifas-Shiman SL, Oken E, et al. Crossing growth percentiles in infancy and risk of obesity in childhood. *Arch Pediatr Adolesc Med.* 2011;165(11):993-998.

17. Tanner JM. *Growth in Adolescence.* 2nd ed. Boston, MA: Blackwell Scientific Publication; 1962.

18. Jonides L, Buschbacher V, Barlow SE. Management of child and adolescent obesity: physiological, emotional, and behavioral assessment. *Pediatrics.* 2002;110:215-221.

19. Parker ED, Sinaiko AR, Kharbanda EO, et al. Change in weight status and development of hypertension. *Pediatrics.* 2016;137(3):e20151662

20. The fourth report on the diagnostic evaluation and treatment of high blood pressure in children and adolescents. National Heart, Lung, and Blood Institute website. www.nhlbi.nih.gov/files/docs/resources/heart/hbp_ped.pdf. Accessed January 8, 2017.

21. Springer SC, Silverstein J, Copeland K, et al. Management of type 2 diabetes mellitus in children and adolescents. *Pediatrics.* 2013:131(2):e648-e684.

22. American Diabetes Association Classification and Diagnosis of Diabetes. In: Standards of Medical of Medical Care in Diabetes—2015. *Diabetes Care* 2015:38(suppl 1):S8-S16.

Chapter 3

The Nutrition Care Process

The Academy of Nutrition and Dietetics developed the Nutrition Care Process (NCP) to improve the quality and consistency of patient/client nutrition care with the goal of improving nutrition care outcomes. It is not intended to standardize nutrition care for patients/clients but to establish a standardized process for providing care.[1-4] This chapter will briefly discuss the NCP, which will be applied to pediatric weight management in Chapters 4 through 9.

The NCP has four steps:

1. Nutrition assessment
2. Nutrition diagnosis
3. Nutrition intervention
4. Nutrition monitoring and evaluation

Patients/clients enter nutrition assessment through screening (discussed in Chapter 2), surveillance system data, or referral, all of which take place outside the NCP.[1]

Step 1: Nutrition Assessment

The purpose of nutrition assessment is to obtain, verify, and interpret data needed to identify nutrition-related problems as well as their causes and significance. During Step 1 of the NCP, the registered dietitian nutritionist (RDN) collects five types of data[1]:

- Food/nutrition-related diet history
- Anthropometric measurements
- Biochemical data, medical tests, and procedures
- Nutrition-focused physical findings
- Client history

Data sources include the following[1]:

- Referring health care providers
- Patient/client interview
- Medical records
- Physical examination and RDN observation
- Team rounds
- Collaborative discussions

In completing the nutrition assessment, the RDN performs the following functions[1]:

- Uses critical thinking skills to determine the appropriate data to collect (ie, relevant versus nonrelevant data)
- Validates collected data
- Organizes data in a meaningful way to make a nutrition diagnosis
- Analyzes and interprets data using evidence-based standards and norms for comparison (eg, the Dietary Reference Intakes or the Academy's Evidence-Based Pediatric Weight Management Nutrition Practice Guidelines)
- Identifies nutrient requirements using reference standards and evidence-based recommendations and guidelines
- Identifies groups or clusters of abnormal or discrepant data

Step 2: Nutrition Diagnosis

In Step 2 of the NCP, the RDN identifies and describes specific nutrition problems based on the results of the nutrition assessment, the RDN's clinical judgment, and the likelihood that treatment/nutrition interventions by an RDN can resolve or improve a nutrition problem. These are not medical diagnoses.[1]

The RDN uses the data collected in the nutrition assessment to identify and label the patient/client's nutrition diagnosis using standardized diagnostic terminology. Each nutrition diagnosis has a reference sheet that includes its definition, possible etiology/causes, and common signs or symptoms identified in the nutrition assessment step.[1]

Following are the three nutrition diagnosis categories[1]:

1. Intake
2. Clinical
3. Behavioral/environmental

The nutrition diagnosis is written in a format known as a PES (problem, etiology, and signs and symptoms) statement.[2,3] A separate PES statement is written for each nutrition diagnosis. The PES statement includes connecting phrases to link the nutrition etiology ("related to") and signs and symptoms ("as evidenced by").

A client may have one or more nutrition diagnoses at one time. In such instances, the nutrition diagnoses are prioritized, an activity that occurs in the next step of the NCP: intervention.[1]

Step 3: Nutrition Intervention

Step 3 of the NCP is defined as purposefully planned actions designed with the intent of changing a nutrition-related behavior, environmental condition, or aspect of health status. Nutrition intervention includes two components: planning and implementation.[1]

Planning

To plan the nutrition intervention, the RDN consults evidence-based practice guidelines, institutional policies and procedures, care maps, and other resources. The Academy's Evidence-Based Nutrition Practice Guidelines provide recommendations for nutrition intervention (www.andeal.org).

During the planning stage, the RDN and the client prioritize nutrition diagnoses based on the following factors[1]:

- Severity of the problems
- Client safety
- Client needs
- Client perceptions of the importance of the problem
- Likelihood that intervention will have a positive impact

Planning also involves working with the client to set short-term (next appointment) and long-term goals. Examples of goals are weight loss, reduction in energy intake, behavior change, increased physical activity, and improvement in knowledge. Goals are carried out in small steps.[1] A gradual approach focusing on one behavior at a time will help build self-efficacy and increase the likelihood of behavior change.[5]

The RDN develops a nutrition prescription that states his or her individualized recommendations. The nutrition prescription concisely states the patient/client's:

- recommended dietary intake of energy or selected foods or nutrients based on current and reference standards and dietary guidelines; and
- health conditions at time of diagnosis.

The RDN links the comparative standards defined in the nutrition assessment step with the client's goals via the nutrition prescription.[1] Planning leads to the selection of specific nutrition interventions and determination of the timing and frequency of nutrition care, including follow-up appointments. Nutrition intervention has four domains:

- Food and/or nutrition delivery
- Nutrition education
- Nutrition counseling
- Coordination of care (eg, collaboration with the pediatrician when the patient has abnormal lipid levels and elevated blood pressure; discussion at pediatric

weight-management team meetings to provide a nutrition update to other members of the team, such as the physician, social worker, and exercise specialist).

Last, the RDN and client define expected outcomes for each nutrition diagnosis. Outcomes are evaluated in Step 4 of the NCP: monitoring and evaluation.

Implementation

Implementation is the action phase of the nutrition intervention and involves the following[1]:

- Ensuring that the intervention plan is implemented as intended
- Communicating the intervention plan to other team members
- Continuing data collection
- Revising the intervention plan when needed based on the client's response and feedback

Step 4: Monitoring and Evaluation

Step 4 of the NCP is monitoring and evaluation. During monitoring, the RDN determines whether the intervention plan was carried out and collects new data related to the desired or expected outcomes selected during the planning phase of the intervention step. Evaluation includes a systematic comparison of the new data with selected criteria to determine progress in achieving desired outcomes.[1]

Criteria for evaluation may include the following[1]:

- Goals
- Nutrition prescription
- Baseline status or status at a previous appointment
- Evidence-based norms and standards

The terminology for nutrition monitoring and evaluation is organized into four domains (categories):

- Food/nutrition-related history outcomes
- Biochemical data, medical tests, and procedure outcomes
- Anthropometric measurement outcomes
- Nutrition-related physical finding outcomes

References

1. Academy of Nutrition and Dietetics. Nutrition Terminology Reference Manual (eNCPT): Dietetics Language for Nutrition Care. http://ncpt.webauthor.com. Accessed March 1, 2016.

2. Lacey K, Pritchett E. Nutrition Care Process and Model: ADA adopts road map to quality care and outcome management. *J Am Diet Assoc.* 2003;103(8):1061-1072.

3. Writing Group of the Nutrition Care Process/Standardized Language Committee. Nutrition Care Process and Model part I: the 2008 update. *J Am Diet Assoc.* 2008;108(7):1113-1117.

4. The Writing Group of the Nutrition Care Process/Standardized Language Committee. Nutrition Care Process part II. Using the International Dietetics and Nutrition Terminology to document the Nutrition Care Process. *J Am Diet Assoc.* 2008;108(8):1287-1293.

5. Shield J, Mullen MC. *The Complete Counseling Kit for Pediatric Weight Management.* Chicago, IL: Academy of Nutrition and Dietetics; 2016.

Chapter 4

Nutrition Assessment and Nutrition Diagnosis

This chapter focuses on the components of a nutrition assessment for children and adolescents who are overweight or obese. In addition, the next step of the Academy of Nutrition and Dietetics Nutrition Care Process (NCP), making a nutrition diagnosis, is also addressed. The NCP and Evidence-Based Pediatric Weight Management Nutrition Practice Guideline recommendations for nutrition assessment and nutrition diagnosis are highlighted throughout the chapter.

A nutrition assessment should be completed after a child or adolescent has been identified as being obese or overweight with health risks (see Chapter 2). For example, a child or adolescent who is overweight and has abnormal lipid levels would need to be assessed for dietary adequacy, including nutrients needed for growth and development, energy intake with special attention to sources of energy and fat intake, and level of physical activity. In addition, a nutrition assessment will help determine areas where changes are needed and areas in which the patient is willing to make changes.

As described in Chapter 3, nutrition assessment is used to identify and evaluate data needed to make a nutrition diagnosis, plan and implement a nutrition intervention, and monitor and evaluate outcomes. Nutrition assessment follows identification of the patient/client by appropriate screening (Chapter 2) or referral. Box 4.1 (see pages 48–49) provides examples of information to be collected in a nutrition assessment of a child or adolescent who is overweight or obese under the different NCP domains. A complete list of these terms, as well as

Box 4.1: Examples of Nutrition Assessment Data Related to Pediatric Overweight and Obesity[1]

Client History

- Personal history: Age, gender, race/ethnicity, grade level, language
- Patient/family-oriented medical history: obesity, diabetes, hyperlipidemia, hypertension
- Social history: Socioeconomic factors

Food/Nutrition-Related History

- Diet experience: Previous diet or nutrition education counseling, previously self-selected diets, dieting attempts
- Mealtime behavior: Whether allowed to select own food, willingness to try new foods
- Eating environments: Eats at designated eating location (ie, does not wander), eats without distractions (eg, watching television/reading)
- Total energy intake
- Fluid/beverage intake: Oral fluid amounts (water, juice, milk, soda)
- Food intake: Amount and type of foods
- Physical activity: Frequency, duration, and intensity of physical activity; television screen time and other sedentary activities

Anthropometrics

- Height/length
- Weight
- Weight change
- Body mass index, body mass index z score
- Growth pattern indexes/percentile ranks

Nutrition-Focused Physical Findings

- Cardiovascular/pulmonary: Shortness of breath
- Digestive: Constipation, heartburn
- Skin: Acanthosis nigricans
- Vital signs: Blood pressure

Continued on next page.

Box 4.1 (cont.): Examples of Nutrition Assessment Data Related to Pediatric Overweight and Obesity[1]

Biomedical Tests/Medical Tests/Procedures

- Lipid profile: Serum cholesterol, high-density lipoprotein cholesterol
- Glucose/endocrine: Glucose, fasting; hemoglobin A1C
- Gastrointestinal profile: Alanine aminotransferase, aspartate aminotransferase
- Vitamin profile: Vitamin D
- Metabolic rate profile: Resting metabolic rate

---

a Nutrition Care Process Terminology (NCPT) code Academy Unique Identifier to be used for data tracking in the electronic medical record, can be found in the electronic NCPT or eNCPT (http:ncpt.webauthor.com).[1]

The information used in the nutrition assessment may be obtained from observations and measurements, the medical record, parent/family interviews, and the referring physician. See Box 4.2 (page 50–51) for various methods for collecting dietary intake data of children and adolescents.[2]

Comparative Standards

Data gathered from a nutrition assessment can be evaluated against comparative standards formulated from evidence-based criteria, relevant norms, and reference standards.[1] For example, data collected from a 24-hour recall or food record can be compared with Estimated Energy Requirements (see Appendix A, page 133) or US Department of Agriculture MyPlate Food Intake Patterns (see Appendix B, page 135). In addition, food record data can be analyzed with a nutrition analysis program to determine macronutrient and micronutrient intake, and then these intake data can be compared with the Dietary Reference Intakes (DRIs). Box 4.3 (see page 52) provides examples of comparative standards.[1]

Box 4.2: Dietary Assessment Methods

24-Hour Recall

Interviewer solicits recall of actual intake in the previous 24 hours from child or caregiver.

Advantages:

- Quick
- Easy to perform
- Provides a snapshot
- Does not require record keeping

Disadvantages:

- May not be reflective of usual intake
- Relies on recollection
- Tends to underestimate intake

3-Day Food Record

Child or caregiver is asked to record actual intake for 3 consecutive days. Client may be provided with a form to record intake or may be asked to keep a diary. Records should include a weekend day to account for differing consumption patterns.

Advantages:

- Data gathered prospectively
- Includes actual (reported) amounts of foods consumed
- Provides a more comprehensive picture of usual intake than a 24-hour recall
- Suitable for computer software

Disadvantages:

- Requires record keeping by child/caregiver

7-Day Food Record

Child or caregiver is asked to record actual intake for 7 consecutive days. Client may be provided with a form to record intake or may be asked to keep a diary.

Advantages:

- Data gathered prospectively
- Provides a more comprehensive picture of usual intake that a 24-hour or 3-day food record
- Suitable for computer software

Continued on next page.

Box 4.2 (cont.): Dietary Assessment Methods

Disadvantages:
- Compliance with keeping the record may be low
- Accuracy may deteriorate over time

Food Frequency Questionnaire (FFQ)

Child or caregiver completes a questionnaire designed to gather data on the frequency and amount of food eaten.

Advantages:
- Decreases time required for the interview if an FFQ is done ahead of time
- Can provide a more complete picture of nutrient adequacy than a 24-hour recall

Disadvantages:
- Difficult to assess unique details of diet
- Overreporting of intake is common

Adapted with permission from the Academy of Nutrition and Dietetics. See reference 4.

Academy of Nutrition and Dietetics Evidence-Based Nutrition Assessment Guidelines

The Academy's Evidence-Based Pediatric Weight Management Nutrition Practice Guideline (PWM NPG)[1] addresses the nutrition management of pediatric overweight and obesity and provides recommendations and ratings for nutrition assessment (see Box 4.4, pages 52–54). The full text of the recommendations is available in the Academy's Evidence Analysis Library.[3] For an explanation of the ratings used in PWM NPG, see pages xi–xiii.

Box 4.3: Terms for Nutrition Assessment/Nutrition Monitoring and Evaluation Comparative Standards[1]

Energy Needs
- Total estimated energy needs
- Methods for estimating energy needs

Macronutrient Needs
- Total fat needs
- Total protein estimated needs
- Total carbohydrate needs
- Total fiber estimated needs

Micronutrient Needs
- Estimated vitamin needs: Individual vitamins
- Estimated mineral needs: Individual minerals

Recommended Body Weight/Body Mass Index/Growth
- Recommended body mass index
- Desired growth pattern

Box 4.4: Evidence-Based Guidelines for Pediatric Weight Management Nutrition Assessment[a]

Foods Associated with Increased Risk of Overweight

Dietary factors that may be associated with overweight and increased total dietary fat and increased consumption of calorically sweetened beverages should be included in the nutrition assessment.

Rating: Strong, Imperative

Food Associated with Decreased Risk of Overweight

Dietary factors that may be associated with a decrease in the risk of overweight and that should be included in the nutrition assessment are increased fruit and vegetable intake.

Rating: Strong, Imperative

Continued on next page.

Box 4.4 (cont.): Evidence-Based Guidelines for Pediatric Weight Management Nutrition Assessment[a]

Assessment: Total Energy Intake and Consumption of 100% Juice

Registered dietitian nutritionists (RDNs) should be aware of the research on the following dietary factors when carrying out a nutrition assessment: reported total energy intake and consumption of 100% fruit juice.

Rating: Fair, Imperative

Assessment: Dairy and Calcium Intake

RDNs should be aware of the observational research indicating that an inadequate intake of dairy and calcium may be related to an increase in the risk of pediatric overweight. Consideration should be given to including dairy and calcium intake as part of the nutrition assessment.

Rating: Fair, Imperative

Family Dietary Behaviors

Child and family dietary behaviors that may be associated with an increase in risk of pediatric overweight and parental restriction of highly palatable foods, consumption of food away from home, increased portion size of meals, and breakfast skipping should be included in the nutrition assessment.

Rating: Fair, Imperative

Family Dietary Behaviors

RDNs should be aware of the research on the following dietary behaviors when carrying out a nutrition assessment: parental encouragement or pressure to eat, parental control over child's dietary intake, meal frequency, snack food intake, and use of food as reward.

Rating: Fair, Imperative

Sedentary Behaviors That Increase the Risk of Pediatric Overweight and Obesity

Sedentary behaviors that may be associated with an increase in the risk of pediatric overweight and should be included in nutrition assessment are excessive television viewing and excessive use of video games.

Rating: Fair, Imperative

Continued on next page.

Nutrition Diagnosis

After the assessment process, data are synthesized to form a nutrition diagnosis. Registered dietitian nutritionists can use the data collected in the nutrition assessment to identify and label the child or adolescent's nutrition diagnosis according to standardized terms. These diagnoses are divided into the following three domains[1]:

- Intake: Too much or too little of a food or nutrient compared with actual or estimated needs
- Clinical: Nutrition problems that relate to the medical or physical conditions
- Behavioral/Environmental: Knowledge, attitude, beliefs, physical environment, access to food, or food safety.

Each diagnosis is written as a problem, etiology, and signs and symptoms (PES) statement. Boxes 4.5 through 4.9 provide sample nutrition diagnoses for pediatric patients who are overweight or obese.[4] Each diagnosis (the "P" in the PES statement) includes at least one sample etiology. The signs and symptoms are identified for each etiology. For more guidance on determining nutrition diagnoses and developing nutrition PES statements, refer to the eNCPT (http://ncpt. webauthor.com).[1]

Box 4.5: Excessive Energy Intake

Etiology	Signs/Symptoms
Food- and nutrition-related knowledge deficit concerning energy intake	Reports intake of large portions of foods/beverages Body mass index ≥95th percentile
Healthful food choices not provided as an option by caregiver or parent	Parent reports that calorically dense foods are less expensive than fruits and vegetables Weight gain in excess of normal growth pattern
Lack of value for behavior change, competing values	Patient/parent reports lack of time to prepare food at home versus eating fast food Weight acceleration from previous growth track

Adapted with permission from the Academy of Nutrition and Dietetics. See reference 4.

Box 4.6: Excessive Oral Intake

Etiology	Signs/Symptoms
Lack of food planning, purchasing, and preparation skills	Patient reports frequent, excessive fast-food or restaurant food intake Weight gain in excess of normal growth patterns
Lack of appetite awareness	Binge-eating patterns Patient reports constant hunger

Adapted with permission from the Academy of Nutrition and Dietetics. See reference 4.

Box 4.7: Altered Nutrition-Related Laboratory Values	
Etiology	**Signs/Symptoms**
Endocrine dysfunction	Elevated plasma glucose and/or hemoglobin A1c levels
	Body mass index for age >95th percentile
Cardiac dysfunction	Elevated serum lipids reported
Liver dysfunction	Increased aspartate aminotransferase and/or alanine aminotransferase
	Weight acceleration from previous growth track

Adapted with permission from the Academy of Nutrition and Dietetics. See reference 4.

Box 4.8: Overweight/Obesity	
Etiology	**Signs/Symptoms**
Excessive energy intake	Report of overconsumption of high-fat and/or caloric-dense foods or beverages
	Body mass index for age >95th percentile
Physical inactivity	Report of infrequent, low-duration, and/or low-intensity physical activity
	Excessive weight gain
Etiology	**Signs/Symptoms**
Not ready for diet/ lifestyle change	Disinterest in applying nutrition-related recommendations
	Weight gain exceeding desired growth pattern

Adapted with permission from the Academy of Nutrition and Dietetics. See reference 4.

Box 4.9: Physical Inactivity	
Etiology	Signs/Symptoms
Lack of available support/role models	Report of patient being home alone while parents are working
Limited access to safe exercise environment	Report of large amounts of sedentary activities
	Parent/patient report that their home is located in an unsafe neighborhood

Adapted with permission from the Academy of Nutrition and Dietetics. See reference 4.

References

1. Academy of Nutrition and Dietetics. Nutrition Terminology Reference Manual (eNCPT): Dietetics Language for Nutrition Care. http://ncpt.webauthor. com. Accessed March 1, 2016.

2. Leonberg BL. *Academy of Nutrition and Dietetics Pocket Guide to Pediatric Nutrition Assessment.* 2nd ed. Chicago, IL: Academy of Nutrition and Dietetics; 2013.

3. Pediatric Weight Management (PWM) Guideline (2015). Evidence Analysis Library website. www.andeal.org/topic.cfm?menu=5296&cat=5632. Accessed March 20, 2016.

4. Pediatric Nutrition Dietetic Practice Group, Kane-Alves V, Tarrant S, eds. *Nutrition Care Process in Pediatric Practice.* Chicago, IL: Academy of Nutrition and Dietetics; 2014.

Chapter 5

Expert Committee Treatment Recommendations

In 2007 the Expert Committee on the Assessment, Prevention, and Treatment of Child and Adolescent Overweight and Obesity published recommendations for the management of overweight and obesity in youth between the ages of 2 and 18 years.[1] The committee, made up of representatives from 15 health professional organizations representing expertise in medicine, nutrition, mental health, epidemiology, and psychology, was convened by the American Medical Association in collaboration with the Department of Health and Human Services Health Resources and Services Administration and the Centers for Disease Control and Prevention.

Pediatric Weight Management Goals

Because childhood and adolescence are times of growth and development, treatment for pediatric overweight and obesity is not as straightforward as treatment for adult overweight and obesity. Therefore, when developing weight-management goals for children between the ages of 2 and 18 years, the Expert Committee considered a youth's age and body mass index (BMI) percentile. Tables 5.1, 5.2, and 5.3 summarize the Expert Committee's age-specific recommendations for weight-management goals for children and adolescents.[1]

Table 5.1: Weight Management Goals for Children Ages 2 to 5 Years[1]

BMI[a] Percentile	Weight Management Goals
85th–94th	Maintain weight until BMI <85th percentile, or reduce rate of weight gain.
≥95th	Maintain weight until BMI <85th percentile. If weight loss occurs, it should not exceed 1 lb/month. If BMI >21 or 22, gradual weight loss (≤1 lb/month) is recommended.

[a] BMI = body mass index.

Table 5.2: Weight Management Goals for Children Ages 6 to 11 Years[1]

BMI[a] Percentile	Weight Management Goals
85th–94th	Maintain weight until BMI <85th percentile, or reduce rate of weight gain.
95th–99th	Maintain weight until BMI <85th percentile, or lose weight (~1 lb/month).
>99th	Lose weight (≤2 lb/week).

[a] BMI = body mass index.

Table 5.3: Weight Management Goals for Children Ages 12 to 18 Years[1]

BMI[a] Percentile	Weight Management Goals
85th–94th	Maintain weight until BMI <85th percentile, or reduce rate of weight gain.
95th–99th	Lose weight (≤2 lb/week) until BMI <85th percentile.
>99th	Lose weight ≤2 lb/week.

[a] BMI = body mass index.

Weight Maintenance

The Institute of Medicine has published sex-specific formulas for calculating Total Energy Expenditure (TEE) for weight maintenance in youth who are overweight or obese. Registered dietitian nutritionists (RDNs) can use TEE as a starting point to determine energy intakes that will result in weight maintenance for children and adolescents who are overweight or obese.[2]

Total Energy Expenditure for Boys

Use the following equation to estimate daily energy needs for weight maintenance in boys between the ages of 3 and 18 years[2]:

$$TEE = 114 - (50.9 \times age\,[y]) + PA\,(19.5 \times weight\,[kg] + 1161.4 \times height\,[m])$$

In this equation, PA is the physical activity coefficient for the individual's estimated physical activity level (PAL; defined as "the ratio of daily total to basal energy expenditure [TEE/BEE]").[4] The following list shows which PA coefficient to use when calculating TEE:

- PA = 1.00 if PAL is ≥ 1.0 and < 1.4 (sedentary)
- PA = 1.12 if PAL is ≥ 1.4 and < 1.6 (low active)
- PA = 1.24 if PAL is ≥ 1.6 and < 1.9 (active)
- PA = 1.45 if PAL is ≥ 1.9 and < 2.5 (very active)

Total Energy Expenditure for Girls

Use the following equation to estimate daily energy needs for weight maintenance in girls between the ages of 3 and 18 years[2]:

$$TEE = 389 - (41.2 \times age\,[y]) + PA \times (15.0 \times weight\,[kg] + 701.6 \times height\,[m])$$

In this equation, PA is the physical activity coefficient for the individual's estimated physical activity level (PAL; defined as "the ratio of total to basal daily energy expenditure [TEE/ BEE]").[2] The following list shows which PA coefficient to use when calculating TEE:

- PA = 1.00 if PAL is ≥ 1.0 and < 1.4 (sedentary)
- PA = 1.18 if PAL is ≥ 1.4 and < 1.6 (low active)
- PA = 1.35 if PAL is ≥ 1.6 and < 1.9 (active)
- PA = 1.60 if PAL is ≥ 1.9 and < 2.5 (very active)

Weight Loss

If weight loss is recommended, goals need to be realistic and individualized. In addition, they should not attempt to fully normalize weight. Approximately 1 lb of weight loss per month may be an appropriate initial goal, with an increase to a maximum weight loss of 2 lb per week as indicated by age and BMI. The long-term weight goal should be a BMI that is less than the 85th percentile for age and sex on the Centers for Disease Control and Prevention growth charts, although some children may be healthy with BMIs in the higher percentile ranges.[1] For youth who are overweight or obese and have serious health complications, such as sleep apnea or pseudotumor cerebri, more aggressive forms of treatment may be necessary (see Chapter 7).

Staged Intervention Approach for Treatment

The Expert Committee recommends the use of a staged treatment approach for children between the ages of 2 and 18 years whose BMIs are at or above the 85th percentile.[1] This approach, which incorporates food or nutrient delivery, nutrition education, nutrition counseling, and coordination of nutrition care, involves four treatment stages of increasing intensity:

- Stage 1: Prevention Plus
- Stage 2: Structured Weight Management

- Stage 3: Comprehensive Multidisciplinary Intervention
- Stage 4: Tertiary Care Intervention

RDNs should adapt the timing of the stages according to the individual families as well as the availability of the programs.[1]

Stage 1: Prevention Plus

Stage 1: Prevention Plus interventions focus on basic lifestyle and physical activity habits (see Table 5.4). These interventions can be implemented by the primary care physician, RDN, or other health professional who has some training in pediatric weight-management and behavioral counseling. Monthly follow-up is recommended. If there is no improvement in BMI or weight status after 3 to 6 months, the Expert Committee recommends advancement to Stage 2, structured weight management, or a higher stage based on the patient/family's readiness for change.[1]

Stage 2: Structured Weight Management

Structured weight-management interventions include all of the Stage 1 primary eating and physical activity goals along with a few others that incorporate a more specific eating and physical activity plan (see Table 5.5, page 65). Compared with Stage 1, Stage 2 involves more support and structure to achieve specific behaviors and can be implemented by a primary care physician, RDN, or other health professional highly trained in pediatric weight management and nutrition counseling. Monthly follow-up is recommended. The Expert Committee recommends that if there is no improvement in BMI or weight after 3 to 6 months, the child or adolescent should be advanced to Stage 3.[1]

Table 5.4: Stage 1 (Prevention Plus): Eating and Physical Activity Goals[1]

Topic	Goal	Comments
Fruit and vegetable intake	Consume at least 5 servings/day; ideally 9 servings/day.	Follow USDA age-specific recommendations for daily amounts.[a]
Sugar-sweetened beverages (eg, soft drinks, sport drinks, and punch)	Minimize or eliminate consumption.	Children who drink large amounts of sugar-sweetened beverages will benefit from reducing intake to 1 serving/day.
Screen time (television, computers, video games)	Limit to ≤2 hours/day.	Discourage television in the room where the child/teen sleeps.
Physical activity	Be physically active ≥1 hour/day.	Encourage both unstructured play (particularly for younger children) and structured physical activities (eg, sports, dance, martial arts, bike riding, and walking).
Meal preparation	Have more home-prepared meals than restaurant food.	
Breakfast	Eat breakfast every day.	Encourage consumption of healthy breakfast foods.

Continued on next page.

Table 5.4 (cont.): Stage 1 (Prevention Plus): Eating and Physical Activity Goals[1]

Topic	Goal	Comments
Food restrictions	Allow youth to self-regulate meals. Avoid being overly restrictive.	
Family involvement	Eat as a family at least 5-6 times/week. Involve the whole family in lifestyle changes.	Tailor behavior change strategies to family's cultural values.

[a] For US Department of Agriculture (USDA) recommendations, refer to MyPlate website (www.myplate.gov).

Table 5.5: Stage 2 (Structured Weight Management): Eating and Physical Activity Goals[1]

Topic	Goal	Comments
Food plan/diet	Follow a planned diet or daily eating plan with balanced macronutrients and low–energy-dense foods (foods high in fiber or water content).	Use DRIs to guide macronutrient distribution.[a]
Meal and snack times	Provide structured daily meals/snacks; no food or caloric beverages between meals and snacks.	Eating breakfast, lunch, and dinner and one or two planned snacks is suggested.
Screen time (television, computers, video games)	Limit to ≤1 hour/day.	
Physical activity	Schedule ≥1 hour/day.	Include planned and supervised activities or active play.
Self-monitoring	Keep detailed records of eating and physical activity behaviors.	Examples include a log of screen time or 3-day food records.
Behavior reinforcement	Plan rewards/contingency management as reinforcement for achieving targeted behaviors.	

[a] For Dietary Reference Intakes (DRIs), see reference 4.

Stage 3: Comprehensive Multidisciplinary Intervention

Stage 3 increases the intensity of behavior changes, the frequency of visits, and the involvement of specialists. A multidisciplinary obesity care team made up of primary care physicians, RDNs, and other health care workers with experience in pediatric weight management, such as nurses, psychologists, social workers, and exercise physiologists, is recommended at this stage, and more frequent office visits are recommended. Weekly follow-up for a minimum of 8 to 12 weeks seems to be the most beneficial. After 12 weeks, monthly follow-up will help maintain new behaviors. Systematic evaluation of body measurements, diet, and physical activity at baseline and throughout the program should be completed to monitor progress.

See Table 5.6 for additional Stage 3 recommendations.[1]

Stage 4: Tertiary Care Intervention

Stage 4: Tertiary Care Intervention is for youth who are severely obese and have not been successful in Stages 1 through 3. Stage 4 is a very intensive intervention that involves referral to a tertiary weight-management center with comprehensive services. These centers operate under a designed protocol, and interventions may involve medications, very-low-calorie diets, and weight-loss surgery. This level of intervention may be offered to some youth who are severely obese after careful evaluation by a team that specializes in pediatric obesity.[1]

More recent recommendations, including the 2010 US Preventive Services Task Force recommendations,[3] Evidence Analysis Library Guidelines,[4] and Academy of Nutrition and Dietetics position paper on Interventions for the prevention and treatment of pediatric overweight and obesity,[5] support the Expert Committee's staged intervention approach for treatment. According to the Academy's position paper,

Table 5.6: Stage 3 (Comprehensive Multidisciplinary Intervention): Recommendations[1]

Topic	Goal	Comments
Food plan/diet	Follow a planned diet or daily eating plan with balanced macronutrients and low–energy-dense foods (foods high in fiber or water content).	Use DRIs to guide macronutrient distribution.[a]
Meal and snack times	Provide structured daily meals/snacks; no food or caloric beverages between meals and snacks.	Eating breakfast, lunch, and dinner and one or two planned snacks is suggested.
Screen time (television, computers, video games)	Limit to ≤1 hour/day.	
Physical activity	Schedule ≥1 hour/day.	Include planned and supervised activities or active play.
Behavior modification	Offer structured behavior modification program with emphasis on self-monitoring, short-term goal setting for diet and physical activity, and rewards/contingency management.	Program should include parents if child is younger than 12 years.
Home environment	Offer training to parents to improve home environment.	

[a] For Dietary Reference Intakes (DRIs), see reference 4.

prevention and treatment for pediatric overweight and obesity can be divided into different intervention approaches,
including primary prevention, secondary prevention, and tertiary prevention (See Table 5.7). Primary prevention includes
interventions that emphasize healthful eating, physical activity, and other health-related activities targeted to the entire
population. Secondary prevention refers to more structured
interventions and strategies to help children who are already
overweight or obese. Tertiary prevention interventions provide the most intensive and comprehensive treatments for
youth who are overweight or obese. Secondary and tertiary
prevention corresponds to the stages approach for treatment
of pediatric obesity recommended by the Expert Committee.[5]

Applying the Expert Committee Recommendations

When treating children and teens who are overweight or
obese, it is very important that RDNs and other health professionals counsel the youth and their families using appropriate
weight-loss goals and staged approach interventions. Table
5.8 (see page 71) summarizes when to apply the Expert Committee's recommended staged intervention approach based
on a youth's age and BMI.[1]

Table 5.7: Definitions of Primary, Secondary, and Tertiary Pediatric Obesity Prevention Compared with the Stage Approach for Treating Pediatric Obesity[5]

	Population	Strategies	Correspondence to Staged Approach for Treatment of Pediatric Obesity	Example
Primary prevention	Population-wide interventions that include youth of all body sizes or weights	Eating and physical-activity messages or programs intended to prevent incidence of overweight/obesity and/or provide a supportive environment for weight maintenance	N/A[a]	School-based health promotion programs for healthy eating and physical activity
Secondary prevention	Overweight or obese youth with no weight-related comorbidities	More structured and involved eating and physical-activity programs intended to help overweight and obese youth obtain a healthy weight; may require medical approval or limited supervision	Stage 1: Prevention Plus Stage 2: Structured Weight Management Stage 3: Comprehensive Multidisciplinary Intervention	Brief motivational interviewing or selected behaviors (eg, decreased consumption of sugar-sweetened beverages) with progression to other stages if warranted

Continued on next page.

Table 5.7 (cont.): Definitions of Primary, Secondary, and Tertiary Pediatric Obesity Prevention Compared with the Stage Approach for Treating Pediatric Obesity[5]

	Population	Strategies	Correspondence to Staged Approach for Treatment of Pediatric Obesity	Example
Tertiary prevention	Overweight or obese youth with comorbidities Severely obese youth	Intensive and comprehensive treatments for overweight or obese youth conducted under medical supervision with a focus on resolving weight-related comorbidities or at least decreasing their severity	Stage 1: Prevention Plus Stage 2: Structured Weight Management Stage 3: Comprehensive Multidisciplinary Intervention Stage 4: Tertiary Care Intervention	Multidisciplinary program offered at a pediatric weight management center, which may include pharmacologic treatment or bariatric surgery

[a] N/A = not applicable.

Reprinted with permission from the Academy of Nutrition and Dietetics. See reference 5.

Table 5.8: Expert Committee Staged Approach to Pediatric Obesity Treatment[1]

Age, y	BMI[a] Percentile for Age and Sex		
	85th–94th	95th–99th	>99th
2–5	Initial: Stage 1 Highest: Stage 2	Initial: Stage 1 Highest: Stage 3	Initial: N/A[b] Highest: N/A
6–11	Initial: Stage 1 Highest: Stage 2	Initial: Stage 1 Highest: Stage 3	Initial: Stages 1–3 Highest: Stage 4 if appropriate
12–19	Initial: Stage 1 Highest: Stage 2	Initial: Stage 1 Highest: Stage 4 if appropriate	Initial: Stages 1–3 Highest: Stage 4 if appropriate

[a] BMI = body mass index.
[b] N/A = not available or not listed.

References

1. Barlow SE. Expert Committee recommendations regarding the prevention, assessment, and treatment of child and adolescent overweight and obesity: summary report. *Pediatrics.* 2007;120(suppl 4):S164-S192.

2. Institute of Medicine. *Dietary Reference Intake for Energy, Carbohydrates, Fat, Fatty Acids, Cholesterol, Protein, and Amino Acids (Macronutrients).* Washington, DC: National Academics Press; 2005.

3. Screening for obesity in children and adolescents. US Preventive Services Task Force website. Published January 2010. www.uspreventiveservicestaskforce. org/Page/Document/UpdateSummaryFinal/obesity -in-children-and-adolescents-screening. Accessed August 20, 2016.

4. Academy of Nutrition and Dietetics. Pediatric Weight Management (PWM) Guideline 2015. www.andeal .org/topic.cfm?menu=5296&cat=5632. Accessed February 20, 2016.

5. Academy of Nutrition and Dietetics. Position of the Academy of Nutrition and Dietetics: interventions for the prevention and treatment of pediatric overweight and obesity. *J Acad Nutr Diet.* 2013;113(10):1375-1394.

Chapter 6

Nutrition Intervention

This chapter covers the nutrition intervention step of the Nutrition Care Process (NCP) and the evidence-based recommendations for nutrition intervention in youths who are overweight or obese issued by the Academy of Nutrition and Dietetics.

Strategies used in developing a nutrition intervention for a child or adolescent who is overweight or obese are based on information obtained from the universal identification or screening, medical and clinical assessment, nutrition and physical activity assessment, nutrition-focused physical exam, and nutrition diagnosis. Recommendations should be individualized, taking into consideration the degree of obesity and health complications associated with overweight or obesity (eg, hypertension, dyslipidemia) as well as any psychological problems (eg, depression, eating disorders). In addition, treatment recommendations must consider the family's readiness to change, family dynamics, financial constraints, and neighborhood characteristics (including access to play areas and grocery stores). Unless all these factors are understood, recommendations for change may not be targeted appropriately.[1-3]

Counseling Goals and Types of Intervention

In counseling children and adolescents who are overweight or obese, the primary goal for registered dietitian nutritionists (RDNs) and other health care providers is to promote more healthful lifestyle behaviors that will help the youth achieve and maintain a healthy body weight.[1-3] The Academy has developed a position regarding the treatment of pediatric obesity and overweight (Box 6.1), which incorporates conclusion statements from the Academy's Childhood Overweight Analysis Work Group.[4] The Work Group's analysis and conclusions are published online at the Academy's Evidence Analysis Library (www.andeal.org).[5]

As discussed in Chapter 5, the Academy of Nutrition and Dietetics has a position paper that supports the Expert Committee's staged intervention approach for treatment.[4]

Box 6.1: Academy of Nutrition and Dietetics Position Statement on Interventions for the Prevention and Treatment of Pediatric Overweight and Obesity[4]

It is the position of the Academy of Nutrition and Dietetics that prevention and treatment of pediatric overweight and obesity requires systems-level approaches that include the skills of registered dietitian nutritionists, as well as consistent and integrated messages and environmental support across all sectors of society to achieve sustained dietary and physical activity behavior change.

Using the Nutrition Care Process

As discussed in Chapter 3, nutrition intervention is the third step of the NCP. The purpose of the nutrition intervention is to resolve the identified nutrition problem by planning and implementing appropriate interventions tailored to the needs of the child or adolescent and his or her family.[5,6] Box 6.2 lists example nutrition intervention terms. Nutrition intervention strategies are designed to change nutrition-related knowledge or behavior, environmental conditions, and access to supportive care or service. Nutrition intervention goals provide the basis for measuring progress and monitoring goals.[6,7]

Standardized Nutrition Intervention Language

The NCP nutrition intervention is divided into four domains[6]:

1. Food and/or nutrient delivery
2. Nutrition education

3. Nutrition counseling
4. Coordination of care

Box 6.2: Nutrition Intervention Terms

Food and/or Nutrient Delivery

- Meals and snacks: General healthful diet
- Meals and snacks: Modify distribution, type, or amount of food and nutrients within meals or at a specified time
- Meals and snacks: Specific foods/beverages or groups
- Vitamin and mineral supplements: Calcium

Nutrition Education

- Initial/brief nutrition education: Purpose of nutrition education
- Initial/brief nutrition education: Priority modifications
- Comprehensive nutrition education: Purpose of nutrition education
- Comprehensive nutrition education: Recommended modifications
- Nutrition counseling theoretical basis/approach: Cognitive-behavioral theory
- Theoretical basis/approach health belief model
- Strategies: Motivational interviewing
- Strategies: Goal setting
- Strategies: Self monitoring

Coordination of Nutrition Care

- Coordination of other care during nutrition care: Team meeting
- Coordination of other care during nutrition care: Collaboration/referral to other providers
- Coordination of care during nutrition care: Referral to community agencies/programs

Adapted with permission from the Academy of Nutrition and Dietetics. See reference 6.

Nutrition Prescription

The RDN develops a nutrition prescription, which is the child or adolescent's individualized recommended dietary intake of energy and selected food or nutrients based on current reference standards and dietary guidelines. The nutrition prescription is not always given to the parent or patient but is used to guide the clinician. The exact specification of nutrients and energy in the nutrition prescription is often translated into a specific eating plan. In addition, the nutrition prescription takes into consideration the patient's health condition and nutrition diagnosis (see Chapter 4).[6,8]

Following is an example of a nutrition prescription: The patient requires a balanced hypocaloric diet of 1,250 kcal/day with 45% to 65% of energy from carbohydrate, 10% to 35% of energy from protein, and 20% to 35% of energy from fat to achieve a healthier weight or to promote weight stabilization.[8]

Evidence-Based Guidelines

As discussed in Chapter 4, the purpose of the Academy's Evidence-Based Pediatric Weight Management Nutrition Practice Guideline (PWM NPG) is to provide evidence-based recommendations for nutrition management of overweight and obesity in children and adolescents. Box 6.3 provides the current recommendations and ratings for the PWM NPG.[5] Refer to pages xi–xiii for the Academy's ratings for recommendations.

Box 6.3: Evidence-Based Guidelines for Pediatric Weight Management Nutrition Intervention[a]

RDN[b] in Multicomponent Pediatric Weight Management Interventions

An RDN should be an integral part of multicomponent pediatric weight-management interventions. A strong body of research indicates that short-term (6-month) and long-term (2-year) decreases in BMI[c] and BMI z scores for all age categories were more likely to be achieved when an RDN or psychologist/mental health provider was involved in multicomponent weight-management interventions that included diet and nutrition (including MNT[d]), physical activity, and behavioral components.

Rating: Strong, Imperative

Multicomponent Pediatric Weight Management Interventions

When providing pediatric weight management, the RDN should ensure that the multicomponent interventions include diet/nutrition (MNT), physical activity, and behavioral components. A strong body of research indicates that short-term (6-month) and long-term (2-year) decreases in BMI and BMI z scores for all age categories were more likely to be achieved when an RDN or mental health professional was involved in the multicomponent pediatric weight-management interventions that included the three major components.

Rating: Strong Imperative

Family Participation in Multicomponent Pediatric Weight Management Interventions

The RDN should encourage family participation as an integral part of a multicomponent pediatric weight-management intervention for children of all ages, including teens. A strong body of research indicates that family involvement as part of a multicomponent pediatric weight-management intervention is highly consistent with positive weight status outcomes at 6 months and 12 months.

Rating: Strong Imperative

Length of Treatment in Multicomponent Pediatric Weight Management Interventions

The RDN should ensure that the multicomponent pediatric weight-management intervention is at least 6 months in duration.

Continued on next page.

Box 6.3 (cont.): Evidence-Based Guidelines for Pediatric Weight Management Nutrition Intervention[a]

Research indicates that shorter-term (less than 6 months) interventions were not consistently associated with positive weight status at 12 months. At least 6 months of treatment was associated with longer-term positive weight status outcomes, especially when group pediatric weight-management sessions were included and treatment occurred in a clinic.

Rating: Fair Imperative

Treatment Setting in Multicomponent Pediatric Weight Management Interventions

The RDN can provide multicomponent pediatric weight-management interventions within the clinic or outside the clinic setting. Research indicates that positive weight status outcomes occur in either setting, especially when the interventions are multicomponent, include group pediatric weight-management sessions, and have family involvement.

Rating: Fair Imperative

Group Sessions in Multicomponent Pediatric Weight Management Interventions

The RDN can include group sessions and family participation as part of the multicomponent pediatric weight-management interventions. Multicomponent intensive interventions that included group pediatric weight-management sessions and family participation were consistently associated with shorter-term (6-month) and longer-term (12-month) positive weight status outcomes.

Rating: Fair Imperative

Individual Sessions in Multicomponent Pediatric Weight Management Interventions

The RDN can include individual sessions as part of the multicomponent pediatric weight-management intervention. Treatment that relied exclusively on individual pediatric weight-management sessions with or without family participation was associated with shorter-term positive weight status outcomes. Information about the longer-term impact on weight status is mixed.

Rating: Fair Imperative

Continued on next page.

Box 6.3 (cont.): Evidence-Based Guidelines for Pediatric Weight Management Nutrition Intervention[a]

Treating Obesity in Children Ages 2 to 5 years

Weight maintenance is generally recommended in 2- to 5-year-old children who are overweight within a multicomponent weight-management intervention with active participation of a parent or caregiver. Weight loss may be recommended when the child has serious medical complications (see Chapter 7).

Rating: Consensus, Imperative

Nutrition Prescription

A nutrition prescription should be formulated as part of the dietary intervention. The exact specification of nutrients and energy is often included in a specific eating plan. Research shows that when a nutrition prescription is included, improvements in weight status are consistent.

Rating: Strong, Imperative

Energy-Restricted Diets: Children Ages 6 to 12 Years

If energy restriction is appropriate, based on the RDN's professional judgment, then a balanced, macronutrient diet that contains no fewer than 900 kcal per day is recommended to improve weight status in a multicomponent program in children ages 6 to 12 years who are medically monitored.

Rating: Strong, Conditional

Energy-Restricted Diets: Adolescents

If energy restriction is appropriate, based on the RDN's professional judgment, then a balanced macronutrient diet that contains no fewer than 1,200 kcal per day is recommended to improve weight status within a multicomponent pediatric weight-management program in adolescents (ages 13 to 18 years) who are medically monitored.

Rating: Strong, Conditional

Tailor Nutrition Education to Nutrition Prescription

In a multicomponent program, if there is a nutrition diagnosis for food- and nutrition-related knowledge deficit, nutrition education should be tailored to the nutrition prescription.

Rating: Fair, Conditional

Continued on next page.

Box 6.3 (cont.): Evidence-Based Guidelines for Pediatric Weight Management Nutrition Intervention[a]

Fast-Food Meal Frequency in Children and Teens

If a child or teen who is overweight or obese consumes fast-food meals, the RDN should encourage reduction in the frequency of fast-food intake to less than twice a week. Limited evidence in populations aged 8 to 16 years at baseline suggests that higher frequency of fast-food consumption, particularly more than twice a week, is associated with increased adiposity; BMI z score; or risk of obesity during childhood and adolescence and during the transition from adolescence to adulthood.

Rating: Weak Conditional

Nutrition Counseling

Nutrition counseling, delivered by an RDN (which is inclusive of goal setting, self-monitoring, stimulus control, problem solving, contingency management, cognitive restructuring, use of incentives and rewards, and social supports) should be part of behavior therapy in a multicomponent pediatric weight-management program.

Rating: Consensus, Imperative

Weight Goals

Weight goals should be individualized to the child. Because of growth occurring within children and adolescents, the goal of weight management may be weight stabilization rather than weight loss (see Chapter 5 for Expert Committee recommendations).

Rating: Consensus, Imperative

Coordination of Care

The RDN should collaborate with members of the health care team to plan and implement strategies.

Rating: Consensus, Imperative

Decreasing Sedentary Behaviors

The RDN should counsel the child or teen to reduce or limit sedentary activities. Intervention research indicates that reducing sedentary activities may have short-term and long-term benefits in terms of pediatric obesity.

Rating: Fair, Imperative

Continued on next page.

Box 6.3 (cont.): Evidence-Based Guidelines for Pediatric Weight Management Nutrition Intervention[a]

Decreasing Sedentary Behaviors: Adolescents

Adolescents should be counseled to reduce or limit sedentary activities. Limited intervention research indicates that reducing sedentary activities may have short-term benefits in managing pediatric obesity.

Rating: Weak, Imperative

---

[a] For an explanation of the ratings, refer to pages xi-xiii.

[b] RDN = registered dietitian nutritionist

[c] BMI = body mass index

[d] MNT = medical nutrition therapy

[e] see Chapter 8

Reprinted with permission from the Academy of Nutrition and Dietetics. See reference 5.

References

1. Barlow SE. Expert Committee recommendations regarding the prevention, assessment, and treatment of child and adolescent overweight and obesity: summary report. *Pediatrics*. 2007;120(suppl 4);S164-S192.

2. Spear BA, Barlow SE, Ervin C, et al. Recommendations for treatment of child and adolescent overweight and obesity. *Pediatrics*. 2007;120(suppl 4):S254-S287.

3. Shield J, Mullen MC. *The Complete Counseling Kit for Pediatric Weight Management*. Chicago, IL: Academy of Nutrition and Dietetics; 2016.

4. Hoelscher DM, Kirk S, Ritchie L, Cunningham-Sabo L; Academy Positions Committee. Position of the Academy of Nutrition and Dietetics: interventions for the prevention and treatment of pediatric overweight and obesity. *J Acad Nutr Diet*. 2013;113(10):1375-1394.

5. Pediatric Weight Management (PWM) Guideline (2015). Evidence Analysis Library website. www.andeal.org/topic.cfm?menu=5296&cat=5632. Accessed March 20, 2016

6. Academy of Nutrition and Dietetics. Nutrition Terminology Reference Manual (eNCPT): Dietetics Language for Nutrition Care. http://ncpt.webauthor .com. Accessed March 1, 2016.

7. Pediatric Nutrition Dietetic Practice Group, Kane-Alves V, Tarrant S, eds. *Nutrition Care Process in Pediatric Practice*. Chicago, IL: Academy of Nutrition and Dietetics; 2014.

8. Recommendations summary. Evidence Analysis Library website. http://andeal.org/template.cfm ?template=guide_summary&key=1280. Accessed March 15, 2016.

Chapter 7

Intensive Interventions for Children and Adolescents Who Are Obese

Children and adolescents who are severely obese and have acute complications, such as pseudotumor cerebri, sleep apnea, obesity hypoventilation syndrome, or orthopedic problems, require more intensive treatment involving a multidisciplinary team.[1-3] In addition to nutrition intervention, individual and family lifestyle modification/behavioral therapy as well as close medical supervision are indicated for this population. Altered macronutrient diets have been explored for use with children and adolescents who are obese. For adolescents, weight-loss medication or weight-loss surgery may be an option. This level of treatment corresponds with the Stage 4: Tertiary Care Intervention of the Expert Committee on the Assessment, Prevention, and Treatment of Child and Adolescent Overweight and Obesity[1,2] (see Chapter 5).

The Expert Committee has the following recommendations for tertiary care intervention:

- Interventions should occur in pediatric weight-management centers that provide comprehensive services.
- The multidisciplinary team should have expertise in childhood obesity and its comorbidities, and patient care should be provided by a physician or nurse practitioner, registered dietitian nutritionist, behavioral counselor, and exercise specialist.
- Standard protocols should be used, and the patients should be evaluated for (1) age and degree of obesity; (2) motivation and emotional readiness to commit to making lifestyle changes; (3) previous efforts in weight control; and (4) family support. These evaluations should focus on the physical and emotional effects of the treatment.

- Unfortunately, some patients who are appropriate candidates for tertiary care intervention may not have access because the programs are not available in their area or their insurance does not cover this type of treatment.

Altered Macronutrient Diets

See Box 7.1 for the Academy's Evidence-Based Pediatric Weight Management Nutrition Practice Guideline (PWM NPG) recommendations for altered macronutrient diets.[4] For an explanation of the ratings, refer to pages xi–xiii.

Weight-Loss Medications

As discussed throughout this book, the focus of pediatric obesity treatment is lifestyle management that incorporates nutrition intervention, physical activity, and behavioral interventions. However, the following weight-loss drug has been approved by the US Food and Drug Administration (FDA) for use with pediatric patients[3]:

- Orlistat (Xenical; Roche Laboratories; www.xenical. com): The drug causes fat malabsorption by inhibiting enteric lipase and has been shown to lead to less weight gain than diet and exercise alone. It is approved for youth with obesity who are age 12 years and older.

Medication should only be used with pediatric patients when incorporated into a multicomponent program.[1,2] See Box 7.2 (page 86) for PWM NPG recommendations.[4]

Weight-Loss Surgery

Weight-loss surgery is a possible option for adolescents who are severely obese and meet a specific selection criterion for adolescent candidates for bariatric surgery (see Box 7.3, page 87–88).[1,5,6] Weight-loss surgery generally results in substantial weight loss and improvements in medical conditions.[5-7]

Box 7.1: Evidence-Based Guidelines: Altered Macronutrient Diets[a]

Very-Low-Carbohydrate Diet: Adolescents

If a very-low-carbohydrate diet is selected for use in adolescents, then it is recommended for short-term (up to 12 weeks) use. However, due to lack of evidence, it is not recommended for long-term treatment of pediatric obesity.

Rating: Weak, Conditional

Protein-Sparing Modified-Fast Diets, Short-Term Treatment

If children or adolescents weigh more than 120% of ideal body weight, have serious medical complications, and would benefit from rapid weight loss, then a protein-sparing modified-fast diet could be used in a short-term intervention (typically 10 weeks) under the supervision of a multidisciplinary team of health care providers who specialize in pediatric obesity.

Rating: Weak, Conditional

Protein-Sparing Modified-Fast Diets, Long-Term Treatment

The protein-sparing modified-fast diet is not recommended for long-term weight management for obesity in children or adolescents. Few well-designed studies support the use of this intervention for longer than 10 weeks.

Rating: Weak, Imperative

Very-Low-Fat Diet

Use of a very-low-fat diet (less than 20% of total daily energy) is not recommended for pediatric weight management. The efficacy of a very-low-fat diet in the treatment of pediatric obesity has not been studied.

Rating: Insufficient Evidence, Imperative

---

[a] For an explanation of the ratings, refer to pages xi–xiii.

Reprinted with permission from the Academy of Nutrition and Dietetics. See reference 4.

Box 7.2: Evidence-Based Guidelines: Weight-Loss Medications[a]

Collaboration With Health Care Team

The registered dietitian nutritionist should collaborate with the health care team regarding the use of weight-loss medications as an adjunct therapy within a multicomponent pediatric weight-management program for adolescents. Clinical outcomes are likely to be enhanced with the participation of a registered dietitian nutritionist.

Rating: Consensus, Imperative

Weight-Loss Medication

If a weight-loss medication is selected as an adjunct therapy, then an over-the-counter or prescription gastrointestinal lipase inhibitor (eg, orlistat), approved by the US Food and Drug Administration for use in adolescents, may be recommended to treat adolescents participating in a multicomponent pediatric weight-management program.

Rating: Fair, Conditional

---

[a] For an explanation of the ratings, refer to pages xi–xiii.

Reprinted with permission from the Academy of Nutrition and Dietetics. See reference 4.

However, perioperative risks, postprocedure nutritional risks, and the necessity of lifelong commitment to altered eating make this approach unattractive or inappropriate for many adolescents. Box 7.4 (see page 88) lists current recommendations regarding types of weight-loss surgery for adolescents.[5,6] Box 7.5 (see page 88) summarizes PWM NPG recommendations.[4] Refer also to the second edition of *Best Practice Guidelines by the American Society for Metabolic and Bariatric Surgery*[5] and *The Academy of Nutrition and Dietetics Pocket Guide to Bariatric Surgery*,[6] which provide a more in-depth discussion about adolescent clients and weight-loss surgery.

Box 7.3: Recommended Selection Criteria for Adolescent Weight-Loss Surgery[6]

Health Status

- Body mass index ≥ 35 with a serious obesity-related medical condition (eg, type 2 diabetes, moderate or severe obstructive sleep apnea, pseudotumor cerebri, or severe steatohepatitis)
- Body mass index ≥ 40 plus a minor comorbidity (hypertension, dyslipidemia, insulin resistance, glucose intolerance)
- Physical maturity (Tanner stage 4 or 5, age > 13 years for girls and > 15 years for boys; exceptions may be made for less mature patients with severe comorbidities

Other Selection Criteria

- Patient has a history of failure at organized weight-loss attempts lasting 6 months or longer
- Patient has demonstrated commitment to comprehensive medical and psychological evaluations before and after bariatric surgery
- Patient has demonstrated commitment to comprehensive medical and physiological evaluations before and after bariatric surgery
- Patient is capable of and willing to adhere to postoperative nutrition guidelines
- Patient is capable of making his or her own decisions
- Patient has a supportive family environment
- Patient agrees to avoid pregnancy for at least 18 months postoperatively
- Parents and adolescent patients provide informed consent to surgery

Contraindications

- Current lactation or pregnancy
- Active substance abuse
- Inadequate social/family support
- Medically correctable cause of obesity
- Unwillingness or inability to fully comprehend the surgical procedure and its consequences, such as lifelong medical surveillance

Continued on next page.

Box 7.3 (cont.): Recommended Selection Criteria for Adolescent Weight-Loss Surgery[6]

- Medical, psychiatric, or cognitive condition affecting patient's ability to adhere to the postoperative diet or medical regimens

Adapted with permission from the Academy of Nutrition and Dietetics. See reference 6.

Box 7.4: Recommendations for Types of Weight-Loss Surgery for Adolescents[5]

- The most common procedures performed in adolescents are Roux-en-Y gastric bypass (RYGB), laparoscopic adjustable gastric banding (LAGB), and sleeve gastrectomy.
- While LAGB is not approved by the US Food and Drug Administration for individuals younger than 18 years, studies have shown that the procedure is effective and safe in adolescents and adults
- Studies have shown that at the 1-year follow-up, weight loss for adolescents who underwent RYGB is at least double that of adolescent patients who underwent LAGB.

Box 7.5: Evidence-Based Guidelines: Weight-Loss Surgery[a,4]

Weight-Loss Surgery

Registered dietitian nutritionists should collaborate with other members of the health care team regarding the appropriateness of weight-loss surgery for adolescents who are severely obese, have not achieved weight-loss goals with less invasive weight-loss methods, and have not met specified criteria. Research indicates that for a subset of adolescents who meet the recommended criteria, weight-loss surgery may be effective in bringing about significant short-term and long-term weight loss.

Rating: Consensus, Imperative

[a] For an explanation of the ratings, refer to pages xi–xiii.

References

1. Barlow SE. Expert Committee recommendations regarding the prevention, assessment, and treatment of child and adolescent overweight and obesity: summary report. *Pediatrics.* 2007;120(suppl 4):S164-S192.

2. Spear BA, Barlow SE, Ervin C, et al. Recommendations for treatment of child and adolescent overweight and obesity. *Pediatrics.* 2007;120(suppl 4):S254-S287.

3. Kelly AS, Barlow SE, Rao G, Ing TH, Hayman LL, Steinberger J, et al. for the American Heart Association Atherosclerosis, Hypertension, and Obesity in the Youth Committee Council on Cardiovascular Disease in the Young, Council on Nutrition, Physical Activity and Metabolism, and Council on Clinical Cardiology. Severe obesity in children and adolescents: identification, associated health risks, and treatment approaches: a scientific statement from the American Heart Association. *Circulation.* 2013;128(15):1689-1712.

4. Pediatric Weight Management (PWM) Guideline (2015). Evidence Analysis Library website. www.andeal.org/topic.cfm?menu=5296&cat=5632. Accessed February 20, 2016.

5. Michalsky M, Reichard K, Inge T, Pratt K, Lenders C. ASMBS pediatric committee practice guidelines. *Surg Obes Relat Dis.* 2012;8(1):1-7.

6. Weight Management Dietetic Practice Group , Cummings S, Isom KA. *Academy of Nutrition and Dietetics Pocket Guide to Bariatric Surgery.* Chicago, IL: Academy of Nutrition and Dietetics; 2015.

7. Inge TH, Courcoulas AP, Jenkins TH, et al. Weight loss and health status 3 years after bariatric surgery in adolescents. *N Engl J Med.* 2016:374(2);113-123.

Chapter 8

Counseling and Behavior Change Strategies

To successfully treat and prevent pediatric overweight and obesity, health care professionals must address not only diet and physical activity but also behavior change.[1-6] There is good evidence (Evidence Grade I) to support behavioral counseling as part of a multicomponent, family-based group intervention for reducing overweight and obesity in school-age children but less evidence (Evidence Grade II) showing the efficacy of behavioral counseling for treating overweight or obesity in teens.[7] (Refer to pages vi–vii for information about the evidence ratings.)

When a child or adolescent and his or her family are ready to make lifestyle modifications, behavior-change strategies should be used to help them. People are not ready to make lifestyle changes until they think it is important and have confidence they can do it. Important components of behavioral counseling for children and teens who are overweight or obese include the following[1-6]:

- Provide nutrition education on lifestyle behaviors and guidance on physical activity and their relation to chronic disease.
- Adapt the home/school environment to help the child or teen make wise food choices.
- Encourage self-monitoring.
- Motivate change by modeling behaviors and contracting.

This chapter addresses evidence-based nutrition counseling considerations, theories and models, and strategies shown to be effective in the pediatric population.

Counseling Considerations for Children and Teens

The Academy of Nutrition and Dietetics Nutrition Counseling Evidence Analysis Library defines *nutrition counseling* as "a supportive process, characterized by a collaborative counselor-patient/client relationship, to set priorities, establish goals, and create individualized action plans that acknowledge and foster responsibility for self-care to treat an existing condition and promote health."[8,9] Compared with adults, children and teens who are overweight or obese present registered dietitian nutritionists (RDNs) with unique counseling challenges that must be addressed to ensure successful weight management. Some of these counseling challenges include the following:

- Who should receive the counseling?
- What type of counseling format works best?
- How should the counseling environment be structured?
- Are there any cultural or ethnic factors to consider?

The following sections summarize how RDNs can address these challenges using current evidence (when available) on counseling children and teens who are overweight or obese and the Academy's Evidence-Based Pediatric Weight Management Nutrition Practice Guideline (PWM NPG).[7]

Family Participation in Counseling

Whereas most adults who are overweight or obese are able to identify and express their dietary and physical activity concerns, this is not the case with children and teens. Therefore, when counseling youth who are overweight, it may be necessary to include parents and adult caregivers.[10] See Box 8.1 (page 92) for the PWM NPG recommendations about family participation in treating obesity in children and adolescents.[7] (Refer to pages xi–xiii for information about the evidence ratings.)

Box 8.1: Evidence-Based Guidelines: Family Participation in Counseling[a]

Family Participation in Multicomponent Pediatric Weight-Management Interventions

The registered dietitian nutritionist should encourage family participation as an integral part of a multicomponent pediatric weight-management intervention for children of all ages, including teens. A strong body of research indicates that family involvement as part of a multicomponent pediatric weight-management intervention is highly consistent with positive weigh-status outcomes at 6 months and 12 months.

   Rating: Strong/Imperative

---

[a] For an explanation of the ratings, refer to pages xi-xiii.

Reprinted with permission from the Academy of Nutrition and Dietetics. See reference 6.

Counseling Setting and Format

In addition to considering who should be counseled, the setting (within clinic versus outside clinic) and format (individual counseling versus group counseling; counseling the parent with or without the child) must also be considered. The PWM NPG recommends family-based counseling for children of all ages in multicomponent pediatric weight-management interventions (see Box 8.2 and Box 8.3 [pages 93 and 94]).

Counseling Environment

The physical surrounding in which the counseling takes place can play a key role in creating a positive learning experience. The RDN should strive to provide a physical environment that will facilitate the counseling experience for both the child and the parent.[10]

Older adolescents are usually comfortable being counseled in an adult environment; however, for younger children it is recommended that the counseling take place in playrooms

---

Box 8.2: Evidence-Based Guidelines: Family-Based Counseling[a]

Treatment Setting in Multicomponent Pediatric Weight-Management Interventions

A registered dietitian nutritionist can provide multicomponent pediatric weight-management interventions within or outside a clinic setting. Research indicates that positive weight-status outcomes occur in either setting, especially when the interventions are multicomponent, include group pediatric weight-management sessions, and involve the family.

Rating: Fair/Imperative

---

[a] For an explanation of the ratings, refer to pages xi-xiii.

Reprinted with permission from the Academy of Nutrition and Dietetics. See reference 6.

---

or counseling rooms specifically designed for them. To help direct a child's attention to items of interest that are age appropriate, the room should be divided by age or developmental level. Consider the following key elements[10]:

- Provide comfortable chairs and tables of sizes suitable for the age, and possibly very large weight, of the children being seen.
- Have oversized or armless chairs to accommodate parents who are overweight or obese.
- Stock the waiting area with age-appropriate books, especially those illustrating nutrition and physical fitness concepts.
- Keep paper and drawing material handy for teaching and for entertaining children while talking with parents/caregivers.
- Hang culturally sensitive posters or pictures that appeal to children.
- Display food models representing recommended portion sizes.
- Ensure that the counseling room is private so the child and family feel comfortable discussing sensitive issues.

Group Sessions in Multicomponent Pediatric Weight-Management Interventions

A registered dietitian nutritionist can include group sessions and family participation as part of the multicomponent pediatric weight-management interventions. Multicomponent intensive interventions that included group pediatric weight-management sessions and family participation were consistently associated with shorter-term (6-month) and longer-term (12-month) positive weight-status outcomes.

Rating: Fair/Imperative

Individual Sessions in Multicomponent Pediatric Weight-Management Interventions

A registered dietitian nutritionist can include individual sessions as part of the multicomponent pediatric weight-management intervention. Treatment that relied exclusively on individual pediatric weight-management sessions with or without family participation was associated with shorter-term positive weight-status outcomes. Information about the longer-term impact on weight status are mixed.

Rating: Fair/Imperative

---

[a] For an explanation of the ratings, refer to pages xi–xiii.

- Have interactive video games available for children to play that involve physical activity or cover child-friendly nutrition topics (see www.choosemyplate.gov).
- Have a computer or tablet available to explore web resources and apps.
- Make a calculator available for counseling exercises involving math, such as tracking physical activity minutes, counting daily calories, or doing label-reading activities.

Cultural/Ethnic Considerations

In addition to the individual's developmental, psychological, and behavioral characteristics, counseling recommendations must fit within the context of the family's culture, living environment, and socioeconomic status.[6,11-14] Compared with the US population as a whole, rates of overweight and obesity are higher in certain ethnic minority populations and in children in families of lower socioeconomic status. The most recent National Health and Nutrition Examination Survey data (2011 through 2014) identified substantial differences in obesity rates among racial or ethnic groups.[14] As discussed in Chapter 1, the prevalence of obesity among non-Hispanic Asian youth (8.9%) was lower than that for non-Hispanic white (14.7%), non-Hispanic black (19.5%), and Hispanic (21.9%) youth.[14]

Counselors must take culturally sensitive and appropriate approaches when working with youth who are overweight or obese. Cultural norms, values, and attitudes strongly influence eating, activity, and perceptions of weight and health.[6,11-13] For example, African American parents and Hispanic parents often perceive elevated body weight in their children as normal or healthy and might be offended if a health professional refers to their child as obese.[14] Low-income families generally have less access to healthy food choices and opportunities for physical activity. Many are lacking nearby retail stores that provide healthy, affordable foods. At the same time, many low-income communities lack or have restricted access to sidewalks, green spaces, parks, and recreation centers perceived as safe; all of these are possible barriers to physical activity. As more is learned about obesogenic environments, it is important for the counselor to recognize these limitations and help the family identify resources and strategies to obtain healthy foods within their budget and get daily physical activity.[15,16] Schools can be a great resource to provide healthful meals. It is important for the RDN to work with schools to provide healthier options.

In some cases (with documentation of medical necessity from a referring physician), an RDN can help direct meal choices, especially in the younger grades.

Numerous resources on tailoring counseling approaches for specific cultures and economic groups are available from the federal government and can be located by searching the nutrition.gov website (www.nutrition.gov).

Nutrition Counseling Theories and Models

Nutrition counseling theories and models are used to design and implement nutrition interventions. The Academy of Nutrition and Dietetics Nutrition Counseling Evidence Analysis Project has explored the evidence of three theories and models as they relate to weight management in adults.[9] However, the use of these theories and models in the weight management of a pediatric population is only beginning to be explored. Although evidence of their success with children and teens who are overweight is yet to be determined, it is still important for RDNs to be aware of these nutrition counseling theories and models.

Cognitive-Behavioral Therapy

Cognitive-behavioral therapy is based on the assumption that all behavior is learned and is directly related to internal factors (eg, thoughts and thinking patterns) and external factors (eg, environmental stimulus and reinforcement) that are related to the problem behaviors. Application involves use of both cognitive and behavioral change strategies to effect behavior changes.[9]

Transtheoretical Model

The transtheoretical model is a theoretical model of intentional health behavior change that describes a sequence of cognitive (attitudes and intentions) and behavioral steps people take in successful behavior change. The model, developed by Prochaska and DiClemente, is composed of a core concept, known as the Stages of Change; a series of independent variables, known as the processes of change; and outcome measures, including decision balance and self-efficacy. The model has been used to guide development of effective interventions for a variety of health behaviors.[9]

Social Cognitive Theory/Social Learning Theory

Social cognitive theory/social learning theory provides a framework for understanding, predicting, and changing behavior. The theory identifies a dynamic, reciprocal relationship among the environment, the person, and behavior. The person can be both an agent for change and a responder to change. This theory emphasizes the importance of observing and modeling behaviors, attitudes, and emotional reactions of others. Determinants of behavior include goals, outcome expectations, and self-efficacy. Reinforcements increase or decrease the likelihood that the behavior will be repeated.[9]

Nutrition Counseling Strategies

Certain nutrition counseling strategies are more likely than others to promote weight management in the pediatric population. No single nutrition counseling strategy works best for every child, teen, or parent/caregiver. In fact, it is wise to use a variety of nutrition counseling strategies to meet individual needs. According to the PWM NPG: "Nutrition counseling strategies should be included as part of a multicomponent pediatric weight-management program. Research shows that when nutrition counseling strategies are included within the context of a multidisciplinary team, weight status and body composition improve."[7]

In addition, the PMW NPG recommends that the following nutrition counseling strategies should be a part of the behavior therapy component of a multicomponent pediatric weight-management program[7]:

- Motivational interviewing
- Goal setting
- Self-monitoring
- Problem solving
- Social support
- Stimulus control
- Cognitive restructuring
- Reinforcement or rewards

The rating for this recommendation is Consensus/Imperative.[7] (See pages xi–xiii for an explanation of this rating.) Boxes 8.4 through 8.11 describe nutrition counseling strategies that are useful in the pediatric population.[9]

Box 8.4: Motivational Interviewing

Motivational interviewing is a directive, client-centered counseling style for eliciting behavior change by helping clients explore and resolve ambivalence. The approach involves selective response to client speech in a way that helps the client resolve ambivalence and move toward change. Four guiding principles underlie this counseling approach:

- Express empathy.
- Develop discrepancy.
- Roll with resistance.
- Support self-efficacy.

The following specific practitioner behaviors are characteristic of the motivational interviewing style:

- Express acceptance and affirmation.
- Elicit and selectively reinforce the client's own self-motivational statements and expressions of problem recognition, concern, desire, intention to change, and ability to change.
- Monitor the client's degree of readiness to change and ensure that encouraging the client to move to the next stage does not generate resistance.
- Affirm the client's freedom of choice and self-direction.

The source of motivation is presumed to reside within the client, and the counselor encourages the client to explore ambivalence and develop self-motivation.

Continued on next page.

Box 8.4 (cont.): Motivational Interviewing

Implementation Tips

Tone of counseling:

- Partnership
- Nonjudgmental
- Empathetic/supportive/encouraging
- Quiet and eliciting

The client does most of the talking, and the counselor guides the client to explore and resolve ambivalence by:

- asking open-ended questions,
- listening reflectively,
- summarizing,
- affirming,
- eliciting self-motivational statements,
- sharing agenda setting/decision making,
- allowing clients to interpret information,
- rolling with resistance rather than confronting,
- building discrepancy,
- eliciting "change talk",
- negotiating a change plan that is initiated by the patient; the plan should start with the patient's agenda, and
- defining the problem as specifically as possible.

Motivational interviewing is best applied in situations in which a patient is not ready, is unwilling, or is ambivalent about changing his or her diet or lifestyle. Motivational interviewing integrates well with the readiness-to-change model to move individuals from the early stages to the action stage of change.

Motivational interviewing is a major paradigm change from the problem-solving type of counseling frequently used by practitioners. Motivational interviewing is not a set of techniques that can be learned quickly but a style or approach to counseling.

Reprinted with permission from the Academy of Nutrition and Dietetics. See reference 17.

Box 8.5: Goal Setting

Goal setting is a collaborative activity between the client and practitioner in which the client reviews all potential activity recommendations and decides what changes he or she will expend effort to implement.

Implementation Tips

- Identify actions appropriate for patients ready to make dietary changes.
- Coach on goal-setting skills.
- Document and track progress toward short-term and long-term goals.
- Probe client about pros and cons of proposed goals.
- Help the client gain the knowledge and skills necessary to succeed.
- Encourage strategies to build confidence (discuss realistic steps and start with easily achievable goals).
- Help clients build a supportive environment.
- Celebrate successes.

Reprinted with permission from the Academy of Nutrition and Dietetics. See reference 17.

Box 8.6: Self-Monitoring

The self-monitoring technique involves keeping a detailed record of behaviors that influence diet and weight. The record may include the following:

- what, when, and how much eaten;
- activities during eating;
- emotions and cognitions related to meals/snacks;
- frequency, duration, and intensity of exercise;
- target nutrient content of foods consumed (ie, calories, fat, fiber);
- the event where eating occurred, thoughts about the event, emotional response, behavioral response;

Continued on next page.

Box 8.6 (cont.): Self-Monitoring

- negative self-talk, replacement thoughts; and
- blood glucose, blood pressure data.

Self-monitoring is associated with improved treatment outcomes..

Implementation Tips

- Provide rationale and instruction for self-monitoring.
- Review and identify patterns.
- Assist with problem solving and goal setting.
- Celebrate successes.
- Recognize that the amount of feedback required typically diminishes as client skill improves.
- Review self-monitoring records with clients to help identify triggers for undesirable eating and barriers to physical activity.

Reprinted with permission from the Academy of Nutrition and Dietetics. See reference 17.

Box 8.7: Problem Solving

Problem-solving techniques help clients identify barriers to achieving goals, implementing solutions, and evaluating the effectiveness of the solutions.

Implementation Tips

Work collaboratively with client to:

- define the problem;
- brainstorm solutions;
- weigh pros/cons of potential solutions;
- select/implement strategy;
- evaluate outcomes; and
- adjust strategy.

Reprinted with permission from the Academy of Nutrition and Dietetics. See reference 17.

Box 8.8: Social Support

Nutrition counseling should encourage increased availability of social support for dietary behavior change. Social support may be generated by an individual's family, church, school, coworkers, health club, or community.

Implementation Tips

A nutrition and dietetics practitioner may assist a client by:

- establishing a collaborative relationship;
- identifying family/community support;
- helping the client develop assertiveness skills;
- using modeling, skill-training, and respondent and operant conditioning;
- utilizing role-play to rehearse ways to respond in different situations;
- conducting education in a group; and
- encouraging family/peer involvement.

Reprinted with permission from the Academy of Nutrition and Dietetics. See reference 17.

Box 8.9: Stimulus Control

Stimulus control (also known as cue management and environmental control) involves identifying and modifying social or environmental cues or triggers to eat, which encourage undesirable behaviors relevant to diet and exercise. In accordance with operant conditioning principles, attention is given to reinforcement and rewards.

Implementation Tips

Help the client identify ways to modify the environment to eliminate triggers. This may include the following:

- Keep food out of sight.
- Remove high-sugar/high-fat snacks from the home.
- Bring lunch to school.
- Establish a rule, such as no eating in the car.

Continued on next page.

Box 8.9 (cont.): Stimulus Control

- Establish criteria for reward for desirable behavior.
- Ensure that reward (reinforcement) is received only if the criteria are met.
- Provide environmental modifications to add positive triggers, for example, setting out a fruit bowl, pedometer, and tennis shoes or putting food records and goal list in a visible spot like the front of a binder.

Reprinted with permission from the Academy of Nutrition and Dietetics. See reference 17.

Box 8.10: Cognitive Restructuring

Techniques used to increase a client's awareness of self-perceptions and beliefs related to diet, weight, and weight-loss expectations.

Implementation Tips

- Self-monitoring and techniques such as the ABC (antecedents, behaviors, consequences) Technique of Irrational Beliefs may help clients become more aware of thoughts that interfere with their ability to meet behavioral goals.
- Help clients replace dysfunctional thoughts with more rationale ones:
  - Challenge "shoulds," "oughts," "musts."
  - Decatastrophize expected outcomes.
  - Confront faulty self-perceptions.
  - Decenter by envisioning another perspective.
- Coach clients on replacing negative self-talk with more positive empowering and affirming statements.

Reprinted with permission from the Academy of Nutrition and Dietetics. See reference 17.

Box 8.11: Reinforcement or Rewards

Reinforcement or rewards (also known as shaping and incentives) is a systematic process by which behaviors can be changed through the use of rewards for specific actions. Rewards may be derived from the client or the provider.

Implementation Tips

- Provide rewards for desired behaviors, for example, attendance, diet progress, consistent self-monitoring.

- Choose rewards such as monetary prizes, gift cards, stickers, books, CDs, or DVDs.

- Help the client determine rewards for achievement.

- Ensure that rewards are not received if progress is not made. Generally, once behavior is consistently performed, rewards are given at less frequent intervals, that is, not every time the behavior is performed. When this level of performance happens, new target behaviors are identified and the reward process starts again with the new desired behavior.

Reprinted with permission from the Academy of Nutrition and Dietetics. See reference 17.

References

1. Barlow SE. Expert Committee recommendations on the assessment, prevention, and treatment of child and adolescent overweight and obesity. *Pediatrics.* 2007;120(suppl 4):S164-S192.

1. Hoelscher DM, Kirk S, Ritchie L, Cunningham-Sabo L; Academy Positions Committee. Position of the Academy of Nutrition and Dietetics: interventions for the prevention and treatment of pediatric overweight and obesity. *J Acad Nutr Diet.* 2013;113(10):1375-1394.

2. Dietz WH, Robinson TN. Overweight in children and adolescents. *N Engl J Med.* 2005;352:2100-2109.

3. Kirk S, Scott BJ, Daniels SR. Pediatric obesity epidemic: treatment options. *J Am Diet Assoc.* 2005;105(5 suppl 1):S44-S51.

4. Spears BA, Barlow SE, Erwin C, et al. Recommendations for treatment of child and adolescent overweight and obesity. *Pediatrics.* 2007;120(suppl 4):S254-S288.

5. Holt K, Wooldridge N, Story M, Sofka D, eds.*Bright Futures: Nutrition.* 3rd ed. Elk Grove Village, IL: American Academy of Pediatrics; 2011. https://bright futures.aap.org/materials-and-tools/nutrition-and -pocket-guide/Pages/default.aspx. Accessed February 11, 2016

6. Pediatric Weight Management (PWM) Guideline (2015). Evidence Analysis Library website. www.andeal.org/topic.cfm?menu=5296&cat=5632. Accessed February 11, 2016.

7. Academy of Nutrition and Dietetics. Nutrition Terminology Reference Manual (eNCPT): Dietetics Language for Nutrition Care. http://ncpt.webauthor. com. Accessed March 1, 2016.

8. Nutrition counseling (NC) systematic review (2007-2008). Evidence Analysis Library website. www.andeal.org/topic.cfm?menu=3151. Accessed February 9, 2016.

9. Shield J, Mullen MC. *The Complete Counseling Kit for Pediatric Weight Management.* Chicago, IL; Academy of Nutrition and Dietetics; 2016.

10. Hudspeth L, Spear B, Lacey H. Weight management: obesity to eating disorders. In: Samour PQ, Helm KK, Lang CE, eds. *Pediatric Nutrition.* 4th ed. Sudbury, MA: Jones and Bartlett; 2012:147-177.

11. Communicating with diverse populations. In: Bauer KD, Liou D, Sokolik CA. *Nutrition Counseling and Education Skills Development.* 2nd ed. Belmont, CA: Wadsworth/Cengage Learning; 2012:218-252.

12. Holli BB, Beto JA. *Nutrition Counseling and Education Skills in Dietetics Professionals*. 4th ed. Philadelphia, PA: Lippincott, Williams & Wilkins; 2012.

13. Ogden CL, Carroll MD, Fryar CD, Flegal KM. Prevalence of obesity among adults and youth: United States, 2011-2014. NCHS Data Brief No. 219, November 2015. www.cdc.gov/nchs/data/databriefs/db219.pdf. Accessed February 20, 2016.

14. Childhood obesity facts. Center for Disease Control and Prevention website. www.cdc.gov/obesity/data/childhood.html. Accessed August 15, 2016.

15. Fisberg M, Maximino P, Kain J, Kovalskys I. Obesogenic environment - intervention opportunities. *J Pediatr (Rio J)*. 2016 May-Jun;92(3 Suppl 1):S30-S39. doi: 10.1016/j.jped.2016.02.007. Epub 2016 Mar 19.

16. Obesity Rates Among Low-Income Preschool Children. Centers for Disease Control and Prevention website. www.cdc.gov/obesity/downloads/pednss factsheet.pdf. Accessed February 11, 2016.

17. Nutrition counseling (NC) aystematic review. Strategy descriptions and application guidance. Evidence Analysis Library website. www.andeal.org/topic.cfm?menu=3151&cat=3946. Accessed February 11, 2016.

Chapter 9

Nutrition Monitoring and Evaluation

As discussed throughout this pocket guide, treatment for children and adolescents who are overweight or obese should focus on improved eating and activity behaviors.[1-3] Follow-up with the child or adolescent is essential to monitor and evaluate behavior changes.

This chapter covers the recommendations for nutrition monitoring and evaluation of pediatric overweight and obesity from the Academy of Nutrition and Dietetics Evidence-Based Pediatric Weight Management Nutrition Practice Guideline (PWM NPG).[4] As mentioned previously, these recommendations are based on the four steps of the Nutrition Care Process (NCP) (see Chapter 3). This chapter also addresses the challenge of follow-up and reimbursement.

The Nutrition Care Process

As discussed in Chapter 3, the fourth step in the Academy's NCP is nutrition monitoring and evaluation, which involves the review of the patient/client's status at a preplanned follow-up and the systematic comparison of current findings with previous status, intervention goals, or a reference standard. In this step, the registered dietitian nutritionist (RDN) completes the following tasks[5]:

- Monitor progress.
- Measure outcomes through nutrition care indicators.
- Evaluate nutrition care indicators against comparative standards.

Box 9.1 provides examples of outcome data that RDNs can obtain when working with children and adolescents who are overweight or obese. The data are arranged by the four domains for nutrition monitoring and evaluation[5,6]:

- Food- and nutrition-related history outcomes
- Biochemical data, medical tests, and procedure outcomes
- Anthropometric measurement outcomes
- Nutrition-focused physical findings

Box 9.1: Examples of Outcome Data for Monitoring and Evaluation[5,6]

Food- and Nutrition-Related History Outcomes

- Amount of food: Per nutrition prescription
- Type of food: Selects appropriately from restaurant or fast-food menu
- Eating environment and location: Eats at designated eating location (ie, does not wander)
- Type of food: Decreases juice and soda intake
- Total energy intake: Limits consumption of food and/or caloric beverages between meals
- Family diet behaviors: Parental restriction of food, consumption of food away from home, portion size at meals, and breakfast consumption
- Family climate factors: Parents' concern about weight, parental support
- Physical activity—duration and frequency: Increases physical activity to 60 minutes each day
- Physical activity—television/screen/media time: Decreases sedentary activity to less than 2 hours each day
- Self-monitoring
- Behavior change goal attainment

Anthropometrics Measurement Outcomes

- Decrease or maintain weight as appropriate
- Decrease in body mass index or body mass index *z* score

Continued on next page.

Box 9.1 (cont.): Examples of Outcome Data for Monitoring and Evaluation[5,6]

Biomedical Data/Medical Tests/Procedures Outcomes

- Improvement in fasting glucose or hemoglobin A1C
- Decrease in cholesterol
- Decrease in low-density lipoprotein cholesterol
- Increase in high-density lipoprotein cholesterol
- Decrease in triglycerides
- Improvement in liver enzymes

Nutrition-Focused Physical Findings Outcomes

- Decrease in blood pressure
- Improvement in shortness of breath
- Constipation no longer a problem
- Decrease in acanthosis nigricans

Standardized Language

NCP Standardized Language combines nutrition assessment and nutrition monitoring terms because the data has substantial overlap in identification and approach. In both steps, data elements are compared with the nutrition prescription, goal(s), or reference standard(s). Most indicators are used for both steps, except those for the Client History domain.[5] See Chapter 4.

Follow-Up Visits with an RDN

If possible, follow-up with an RDN within 1 week to 1 month. Greater frequency of contacts between the client and the RDN may lead to more successful weight loss and maintenance. The Expert Committee on the Assessment, Prevention, and Treatment of Child and Adolescent Overweight and Obesity recommends the following[1,2]:

- Monthly follow-up for clients in Stage 1: Prevention Plus or Stage 2: Structured Weight Management (see Chapter 5 for explanation of the treatment stages).

- Weekly follow-up for a minimum of 8 to 12 weeks, and then monthly follow-up is more appropriate for clients in a Stage 3: Comprehensive Multidisciplinary Intervention.
- If a specific timeframe is not feasible (eg, due to financial or time constraints or travel distance to appointments), the timing of counseling sessions should be adjusted appropriately. In the case of distance, the RDN might consider working with a local RDN for follow-up.

The PWM NPG recommendation for optimal length of treatment for pediatric overweight and obesity is provided in Box 9.2.[4]

Box 9.2: Evidence-Based Recommendation for Optimal Length of Treatment[a]

During the intensive treatment phase, medical nutrition therapy for pediatric obesity should last at least 3 months or until initial weight-management goals are achieved. Because overweight and obesity are chronic, it is critical that a weight-management plan can be implemented after the intensive phase of treatment. A greater frequency of contacts between the patient and RDN may lead to more successful weight loss and maintenance.

Rating: Consensus, Imperative

[a] For an explanation of the evidence rating, refer to pages xi–xiii.

Reprinted with permission from the Academy of Nutrition and Dietetics. See reference 4.

During follow-up visits, RDNs should focus on behavior changes that lead to more healthful eating and physical activity habits, rather than emphasizing change in body weight. For example, RDNs should take time to review food and activity diaries for evidence of behavior change. Motivational interviewing questions can help assess behavior change.[3] See Box 9.3 for some examples of motivational interviewing questions. For more information on behavior change see Chapter 8.

> **Box 9.3: Motivational Interviewing Questions to Assess Behavior Change[3]**
>
> - It sounds like you and your child have been trying to make some lifestyle changes since we met last. Can you tell me about that?
> - We set some goals at the last visit. How do you feel you did in meeting those goals?
> - What new physical activities has your family started since our last visit?
> - It sounds like you have been trying to make some changes but have found that it isn't as easy as you thought. Is that what you are feeling?

Medical Nutrition Therapy and Reimbursement

Follow-up is essential for identifying the benefits of medical nutrition therapy (MNT), a fundamental component of health care coverage. Thorough documentation of patient outcomes (Box 9.1, see pages 108–109) and the effectiveness of MNT in pediatric overweight and obesity affirms the positive impact of MNT and is needed to help expand reimbursement for pediatric obesity/overweight.[3,7] The practice section of the Academy of Nutrition and Dietetics website (www.eatright. org/mnt) has many resources available to assist RDNs with outcomes of MNT.

One challenge facing RDNs who provide nutrition counseling to children and teens who are overweight or obese is the lack of third-party reimbursement, which may limit the frequency of an individual's visits with an RDN.[3] Contact insurance companies regarding their coverage policies for MNT or nutrition counseling. The practice section of the Academy of Nutrition and Dietetics website has many resources available to assist RDNs seeking coverage and reimbursement for nutrition services (www.eatrightpro

.org/resources/practice/getting-paid) as well as resources
related to ICD-10 and Current Procedural Terminology codes
(www.eatrightpro.org/resource/practice/getting-paid/nuts
-and-bolts-of-getting-paid/icd-10-cm). Box 9.4 provides
suggestions about how to help clients/patients obtain MNT
coverage.[7]

Box 9.4: Selected Ways to Help Clients Obtain Medical Nutrition Therapy[7]

Following are ways to help expand coverage for medical nutrition therapy services for children and adolescents who are overweight or obese:

- Assess local coverage provided by insurers. Determine how one insurer is providing nutrition services for registered dietitian nutritionists and try to emulate with other plans.

- Know the child or adolescent's nutrition needs and state those in your goals to policy decision makers.

- Talk to other registered dietitian nutritionists who work with children and teens who are overweight or obese and learn from their experiences.

- Keep abreast of any pending legislation that might support your efforts.

- Arrange to meet with the payer's medical director and other decision makers.

Follow-Up With Client's Pediatrician and Privacy Issues

It is important to provide the child or teen's pediatrician with progress notes regarding the client's progress. The RDN should send a progress note through email or electronic medical records or call the pediatrician to summarize outcomes, such as body mass index changes and eating and physical activity behaviors.[3] The RDN may also need to request a physician referral that indicates the medical necessity for additional nutrition counseling sessions. This may increase the likelihood that the additional MNT visits will qualify for insurance reimbursement. Additionally, the RDN should obtain updates on laboratory values, when available for the client.[1-3] If working as part of a multidisciplinary team, the RDN should also update other team members regarding the child or adolescent's progress. The electronic health record (EHR) serves as a tool for communicating among health care members and a tool to track both progress and outcome measures. Box 9.1 (see pages 108–109) lists possible outcome data to be included in the EHR.

Under the Health Insurance Portability and Accountability Act (HIPAA) regulations, RDNs, as covered entities, are allowed to disclose protected health information for treatment purposes without the patient's authorization.[8] RDNs should create a privacy notice that describes how the RDN will protect client's health information. The notice should be distributed to all patients before the first MNT visit, and the RDN should obtain written acknowledgment from all patients that they have reviewed and have a copy of the practice's privacy notice. Academy members can access a sample HIPAA privacy notice for RDNs in private practice and a sample written acknowledgment confirming receipt of the privacy notice from the Academy of Nutrition and Dietetcs.[9]

Promoting Follow-Up Communication with Clients

To increase follow-up communication when counseling youth who are overweight or obese and their families, RDNs should be flexible and creative. Suggestions for follow-up include the following[3]:

- Schedule sessions to fit the family's schedule.
- Communicate by email, text, phone, mail, or face time in a secure location. Always ensure that HIPAA requirements for electronic communication are met.
- Use communication tools available through My Chart, which offers patients and families personalized and secure online access to portions of the EHR.

- Develop a webpage.
- Researchers are evaluating the use of social media and apps for weight management and health behavior change.[11,12] Provide a list of some apps for healthy eating and physical activity behaviors as well as weight-management tools. The RDN can often share information and patient progress through these apps The Academy of Nutrition and Dietetics provides reviews of apps for both adults and children (www.eatright.org).
- Emphasize the importance of self-monitoring between visits.
- Provide information about community resources and programs.
- Discuss peer support groups

References

1. Barlow SE. Expert Committee recommendations regarding the prevention, assessment, and treatment of child and adolescent overweight and obesity: summary report. *Pediatrics.* 2007;120(suppl 4):S164-S192.

2. Spear BA, Barlow SE, Ervin C, et al. Recommendations for treatment of child and adolescent overweight and obesity. *Pediatrics.* 2007;120(suppl 4):S254-S287.

3. Shield J, Mullen MC. *The Complete Counseling Kit for Pediatric Weight Management.* Chicago, IL: Academy of Nutrition and Dietetics; 2016.

4. Pediatric Weight Management (PWM) Guideline (2015). Evidence Analysis Library website. www.andeal.org/topic.cfm?menu=5296&cat=5632. Accessed March 20, 2016.

5. Academy of Nutrition and Dietetics. Nutrition Terminology Reference Manual (eNCPT): Dietetics Language for Nutrition Care. http://ncpt.webauthor.com. Accessed Accessed March 1, 2016.

6. Pediatric Nutrition Dietetic Practice Group, Kane-Alves V, Tarrant S, eds. *Nutrition Care Process in Pediatric Practice.* Chicago, IL: Academy of Nutrition and Dietetics; 2014.

7. Michael P, Brodney S. Weight management counseling: a guide to understanding coverage, reimbursement and opportunities for registered dietitians. *Weight Management Newsletter.* 2008;5:4-8.

8. HIPAA Frequent Questions. www.hhs.gov/hipaa/for-professionals/faq. US Department of Health and Human Services website. Accessed March 21, 2106.

9. *MNT Practice Tools: Sample HIPAA Privacy Notice for RDs in Private Practice.* Chicago, IL: Academy of Nutrition and Dietetics; 2015.

10. Patrick K, Marshall EP, Kolodziejck JK, et al. Design and implementation of a randomized controlled social and mobile weight loss trial for young adults (project SMART). *Contemp Clin Trials.* 2014; 37(1):10-18.

11. Shoffman DE, Turner McGrievy GT, Jones SJ, Wilcox S. Mobile apps for pediatric obesity prevention and treatment, healthy eating, and physical activity promotion: just fun and games? *Transl Behav Med.* 2013;3(3):320-325.

Chapter 10

Prevention

The previous chapters have discussed the major issues and challenges registered dietitian nutritionists (RDNs) face while working with youth who are overweight or obese and their families. Although much work is being done to determine the best ways to screen, assess, and treat these children and adolescents, prevention remains the most promising solution to this serious health problem.[1-3]

This chapter will provide an overview of the pediatric overweight and obesity prevention recommendations from the Expert Committee on the Assessment, Prevention, and Treatment of Child and Adolescent Overweight and Obesity,[1] the Institute of Medicine (see Box 10.1),[2] the World Health Organization (see Box 10.2),[3] and the Academy of Nutrition and Dietetics Evidence-Based Pediatric Weight Management Nutrition Practice Guideline (PWM NPG).[4]

Box 10.1: Institute of Medicine Recommendations on Pediatric Overweight and Obesity Prevention[2]

The Institute of Medicine released a 2012 report addressing the problem of childhood obesity in the United States, *Accelerating Progress in Obesity Prevention*, which included the following recommendations:

- Make physical activity an integral and routine part of life.
- Create food and beverage environments that ensure healthy food and beverage options are routine, easy choices.
- Market healthy messages about physical activity and nutrition.
- Expand the role of health care providers, insurers, and employers in obesity prevention.
- Make schools a national point for obesity prevention.

> **Box 10.2: World Health Organization Recommendations on Pediatric Overweight and Obesity Prevention[3]**
>
> The World Health Organization's 2016 *Report of the Commission on Ending Childhood Obesity* included the following recommendations:
>
> - Implement comprehensive programs that promote intake of healthy foods and decrease intake of unhealthy foods and sugar-sweetened beverages.
> - Implement comprehensive programs to promote physical activity and reduce sedentary behaviors.
> - Integrate and strengthen guidance for preconception and antenatal care to reduce the risk of childhood obesity.
> - Provide guidance and support for healthy diet, sleep, and physical activity in early childhood.
> - Implement comprehensive programs that promote healthy school environments, health and nutrition literacy, and physical activity among schoolchildren.

Expert Committee Prevention Recommendations

Prevention of pediatric overweight and obesity is the best form of treatment. The Expert Committee recognized this fact in making the primary goal of obesity treatment the improvement of long-term physical health through permanent healthful lifestyle habits. The Expert Committee recommends that physicians and RDNs address the issue of weight with all children at least once per year. If weight issues are present or if the family presents with other nutrition-related concerns the RDN should meet with the patient and family more frequently. Lifestyle factors that should be targeted as part of the assessment include food and nutrient intake, physical activity, and knowledge/beliefs/attitudes about making behavior changes. (See Chapters 2 and 4 for detailed information about obesity risk assessment and nutrition assessment.) As described in the following sections, the Expert Committee recommends a slightly modified form of the Stage 1: Prevention Plus strategy (see Chapter 5) for children ages 2 to 18 years whose body mass index is at or more than the 5th percentile for age and sex and no greater than the 84th percentile.[1]

Improve Dietary Intake and Healthful Eating Behaviors

Please note: The Dietary Reference Intakes and Dietary Guidelines for Americans should be used when applying nutrition-related Expert Committee prevention guidelines to individual youths[2,5,6]:

- Limit the consumption of sugar-sweetened beverages, such as soda, sport drinks, sweetened fruit drinks, and sweetened teas.
- Encourage the consumption of five or more servings of fruits and vegetables per day. Ideally, families should strive for nine servings per day as recommended by the US Department of Agriculture (www.myplate.gov).
- Eat breakfast daily.
- Limit meals at restaurants, particularly fast-food restaurants.
- Encourage family meals in which parents and children eat together—aim for five or six times per week. Parents should take advantage of meal time to serve as healthy role models. In addition, if schedules do not allow for the families to always meet at dinner try breakfast or lunch on the weekends.
- Limit food portion sizes. (US Department of Agriculture recommendations [www.myplate.gov] provide age-appropriate portion sizes for a variety of foods both in common household measures and visually.)
- Eat a diet rich in calcium.
- Eat a diet high in fiber.
- Eat a diet with balanced macronutrients (calories from fat, carbohydrate, and protein) in proportions appropriate for age as recommended in the Dietary Reference Intakes.[4]

- Limit the consumption of energy-dense foods. Energy-dense foods are foods that provide a large amount of calories in a small amount/weight of food (eg, candy, pastries, and snack chips).

Decrease Physical Inactivity

- Limit television and other screen time to no more than 2 hours per day starting when children are 5 years old.
- Remove television and computer screens from children's primary sleeping areas as recommended by the American Academy of Pediatrics.[6]

Increase Physical Activity

- Participate in at least 60 minutes of moderate to vigorous physical activity daily, which can be accumulated throughout the day, as opposed to only single or long bouts.
- Help children and teens identify and participate in physical activities that they find enjoyable.

Public Health Advocacy

As part of a more community-based effort to prevent pediatric obesity, the Expert Committee recommends that organizations for physicians, RDNs, and health professionals advocate that the federal government do the following[1]:

- Increase physical activity at school through intervention programs as early as grade 1 through the end of high school and college as well as by creating school environments that support physical activity overall.
- Support efforts to preserve and enhance parks as areas for physical activity, informing local development initiatives regarding the inclusion of walking and bicycle paths, and promoting families' use of local physical

activity options by making information and suggestions about physical activity alternatives available in
doctors' offices.

Family-Based Initiatives

Finally, the Expert Committee recommends using the following techniques to aid physicians and RDNs who may wish
to support obesity prevention in clinical, school, and community settings[1]:

- Provide prevention interventions to families with parents
  who are overweight or obese or mothers with a history
  of diabetes during pregnancy, even if the children currently have a healthy body mass index. These children
  are at increased risk for developing obesity.

- Discourage a restrictive parenting style that heavily monitors and controls a child's eating, which may lead to a
  disordered eating pattern.

- Encourage an authoritative parenting style regarding a
  child's eating and physical activity. Authoritative parents
  teach and set clear standards for their children; they are
  assertive but not intrusive or too restrictive.

- Stress the importance of parents being positive role models for eating and physical activity.

Evidence-Based Prevention Research

The Academy of Nutrition and Dietetics PWM NPG aligns
with the Expert Committee recommendations on prevention.
The PWM NPG recommendations serve as a framework for
treating pediatric overweight and obesity through interventions with children, adolescents, and their families, and they
also serve as a framework for preventive strategies. Tables
10.1 through 10.5 summarize current evidence on diet, dietary
behaviors, physical activity, parent/child relationship, and

social influences associated with childhood and adolescent overweight and obesity.[4] For detailed information, visit the Evidence Analysis Library (www.andeal.org).

Table 10.1: Food and Nutrient Factors Associated with Pediatric Overweight and Obesity[4]		
Factor	Conclusion	Evidence Grade[a]
Calcium	Low intake of calcium may be associated with increased adiposity.	III: Limited
Dairy	Low intake of dairy may be associated with increased adiposity among children.	III: Limited
Fruit juice	Intake of 100% fruit juice is not associated with increased adiposity in children unless consumed in unusually large quantities.	II: Fair
Fruits and vegetables	Intake of fruits and vegetables is inversely related to adiposity in children.	II: Fair
Sweetened beverages	Intake of calorically sweetened beverages is positively related to adiposity in children.	II: Fair
Dietary fat	Dietary fat intake is associated with higher adiposity in youth.	II: Fair
Total energy intake	Total energy (caloric) intake measured using current dietary assessment tools, which may not accurately assess total energy intake, does not seem to have a strong association with overweight.	II: Fair

[a] For an explanation of the evidence grades, refer to pages xi–xiii.

Table 10.2: Dieting Behavior Factors Associated with Pediatric Overweight and Obesity[a]

Factor	Conclusion	Evidence Grade[a]
Eating frequency	Eating frequency may not be associated with adiposity.	III: Limited
Snacking	Snacking frequency or snack food intake may not be associated with adiposity.	III: Limited
Breakfast skipping	Breakfast skipping may be associated with increased adiposity, particularly among older children and adolescents and for those who are healthy weight (as opposed to those who are already overweight).	III: Limited
Eating out	Consumption of food away from home, particularly at fast-food establishments, may be associated with adiposity, especially among adolescents.	III: Limited
Portion sizes	Increased portion sizes may be associated with adiposity in children.	III: Limited

[a] For an explanation of the evidence grades, refer to pages xi–xiii.

Table 10.3: Physical Activity Factors Associated with Childhood Overweight and Obesity[a]

Factor	Conclusion	Evidence Grade[a]
Television time	Excessive television viewing is associated with increased adiposity in youth.	II: Fair
Video games	Excessive use of video games may be associated with increased adiposity in youth.	III: Limited
Physical activity	Participation in regular physical activity is associated with lower adiposity in youth. This association is stronger in boys than in girls.	II: Fair
Sports activity	Participation in sports may be associated with lower adiposity.	III: Limited

[a] For an explanation of the evidence grades, refer to pages xi–xiii.

Table 10.4: Parent/Child Relationship Associated with Childhood Overweight and Obesity[4]

Factor	Conclusion	Evidence Grade[a]
Parental control	The parental child-feeding practice/style, or parental control over the child's dietary intake, does not seem to be associated with overweight in children.	II: Fair
Parental criticism	Parental concern about a child's weight status may be associated with overweight in children; however, a majority of the research has been conducted among non-Hispanic white girls and may be applicable only to this population.	II: Fair
Pressure to eat	Parental pressure to eat is not associated with increased overweight in children.	II: Fair
Restriction	Parental restriction of highly palatable foods may promote children's desire for such forbidden foods, causing dysregulation of energy intake and over-eating. It seems that this child-feeding practice is associated with overweight in children; however, a majority of the research has been conducted among non-Hispanic white girls and may be applicable only to this population.	II: Fair

Continued on next page.

Table 10.4 (cont.): Parent/Child Relationship Associated with Childhood Overweight and Obesity[a]

Factor	Conclusion	Evidence Grade[a]
Instrumental feeding	Based on limited evidence, the parental child-feeding practices of using food as a reward (instrumental feeding) and emotional feeding, which may be considered a specific type of parental control over a child's dietary intake, do not seem to be associated with overweight in children.	III: Limited
Family functioning	Positive aspects of family functioning, such as family cohesion, expressiveness, democratic style, parental support, and cognitive stimulation at home, may be protective against childhood overweight, whereas other negative aspects of family functioning, such as lack of parental support or overpossessiveness may be associated with overweight among children. At present, however, it is challenging to compare studies because of different constructs used to assess family functioning.	III: Limited

[a] For an explanation of the evidence grades, refer to pages xi–xiii.

Table 10.5: Social Influences Associated with Childhood Overweight and Obesity[a]

Factor	Conclusion	Evidence Grade[a]
Food insecurity	Household food insecurity does not seem to be associated with overweight among children, a finding that may be due in part to the fact that a comprehensive measure of child food insecurity was not used in most studies.	II: Fair
Parental diet attitude	Parental dietary disinhibition and restraint may be related to a higher risk of overweight in children. Parents are likely to exert control over their children's behavior in areas that are important and potentially problematic for themselves; however, these studies have only been conducted among predominantly white, middle-class populations and therefore these results may not be applicable to other populations.	III: Limited

[a] For an explanation of the evidence grades, refer to pages xi–xiii.

Promotion of Physical Activity

The US Surgeon General and the 2010 Dietary Guidelines for Americans recommend that children and adolescents engage in at least 60 minutes of physical activity of at least moderate intensity on most, but preferably all, days. Examples of moderate-intensity aerobic activity or vigorous-intensity activity are provided in Table 10.6 (see pages 128–130).[7,8]

- Several approaches may be used to increase physical activity.[8]
- Children and adolescents should limit screen entertainment time to less than 2 hours per day.[9]
- Limitation of television, video games, and computer games will encourage children to choose other pastimes, most of which will generate more physical activity.[9]
- Increased physical activity may lead to improved strength and fewer injuries.[8]
- Internet/television/video games can be used to promote increased physical activity in cold winter months when playing outside is not an option.[8,9]

Table 10.6: Aerobic, Muscle-Strengthening, and Bone-Strengthening Activities: What Counts?

Type of Physical Activity	Age Group	
	Children	Adolescents
Moderate-intensity aerobic	Active recreation, such as hiking, skateboarding, and rollerblading Bicycle riding Walking to school	Active recreation, such as canoeing, hiking, cross-country skiing, skateboarding, and rollerblading Brisk walking Bicycle riding (stationary or road bike) House and yard work, such as sweeping or pushing a lawnmower Playing games that require catching and throwing, such as baseball, softball, basketball, and volleyball

Continued on next page.

Table 10.6 (cont.): Aerobic, Muscle-Strengthening, and Bone-Strengthening Activities: What Counts?

Type of Physical Activity	Age Group	
	Children	Adolescents
Vigorous-intensity aerobic	Active games involving running and chasing, such as tag Bicycle riding Jumping rope Martial arts, such as karate Running Sports such as ice or field hockey, basketball, swimming, tennis, or gymnastics	Active games involving running and chasing, such as flag football and soccer Bicycle riding Jumping rope Martial arts, such as karate Running Sports such as tennis, ice or field hockey, basketball, and swimming Vigorous dancing Aerobics Cheerleading or gymnastics

Continued on next page.

Table 10.6 (cont.): Aerobic, Muscle-Strengthening, and Bone-Strengthening Activities: What Counts?

Type of Physical Activity	Age Group	
	Children	Adolescents
Muscle strengthening	Games such as tug-of-war Modified push-ups (with knees on the floor) Resistance exercises using body weight or resistance bands Rope or tree climbing Sit-ups Swinging on playground equipment/bars Gymnastics	Games such as tug-of-war Push-ups Resistance exercises with exercise bands, weight machines, or handheld weights Rock-climbing Sit-ups Cheerleading or gymnastics
Bone strengthening	Games such as hopscotch Hopping, skipping, and jumping Jumping rope Running Sports such as gymnastics, basketball, volleyball, and tennis	Hopping, skipping, and jumping Jumping rope Running Sports such as gymnastics, basketball, volleyball, tennis

Adapted with permission from the Centers for Disease Control and Prevention. See reference 7.

References

1. Barlow SE. Expert Committee recommendations regarding the prevention, assessment, and treatment of child and adolescent overweight and obesity: summary report. *Pediatrics.* 2007;120(suppl 4): S164-S192.

2. Institute of Medicine. *Accelerating Progress in Obesity Prevention: Solving the Weight of the Nation.* Washington, DC: National Academies Press; 2012.

3. World Health Organization. *Report of the Commission on Ending Childhood Obesity.* http://apps.who.int/ iris/bitstream/10665/204176/1/9789241510066 _eng.pdf?ua=1. Accessed February 1, 2016.

4. Pediatric Weight Management (PWM) Guideline (2015). Evidence Analysis Library website. www.andeal.org/topic.cfm?menu=5296&cat=5632. Accessed February 20, 2016.

5. Comprehensive Dietary Reference Intake table for vitamins, minerals, and macronutrients; organized by age and gender. Institute of Medicine website. www.nal.usda.gov/fnic/dri-tables-and-application -reports=. Accessed March 16, 2016.

6. US Department of Health and Human Services and US Department of Agriculture. Dietary Guidelines for Americans 2015-2020. 8th ed. http://health.gov /dietaryguidelines/2015/guidelines/. Accessed March 16, 2009.

7. Physical activity for everyone. How much exercise do children need? Centers for Disease Control and Prevention website. www.cdc.gov/physicalactivity /everyone/guidelines/children.html. Updated June 4, 2015. Accessed March 16, 2016.

8. American Academy of Pediatrics. Children, adolescents, and the media. *Pediatrics.* 2013;132(5):958-964. http://pediatrics.aappublications org/content/early/2013/10/24/peds.2013-2656.full.pdf +html. Accessed September 20,2014.

9. US Department of Health and Human Services. *Physical Activity Guidelines for Americans.* Washington, DC: Government Printing Office; 2008.

Appendix A

Dietary Reference Intakes: Estimated Energy Requirements

	Estimated Energy Requirements for Boys and Girls Ages 3 to 18 Years[a]
Age, y	Estimated Energy Requirements, kcal/d
3–8	**Boys:** $108.5 - 61.9 \times \text{Age (y)} + \text{PA}^b \times (26.7 \times \text{Weight [kg]} + 903 \times \text{Height [m]})$ **Girls:** $155.3 - 30.8 \times \text{Age (y)} + \text{PA} \times (10.0 \times \text{Weight [kg]} + 934 \times \text{Height [m]})$
9–18	**Boys:** $113.5 - 61.9 \times \text{Age (y)} + \text{PA} \times (26.7 \times \text{Weight [kg]} + 903 \times \text{Height [m]})$ **Girls:** $160.3 - 30.8 \times \text{Age (y)} + \text{PA} \times (10.0 \times \text{Weight [kg]} + 934 \times \text{Height [m]})$

[a] See Chapter 5 for Total Energy Expenditure (TEE) formulas for weight maintenance in youth who are overweight or obese.

[b] PA = physical activity

From Leonberg, BL. *The Academy of Nutrition and Dietetics Pocket Guide to Pediatric Nutrition Assessment.* 2nd ed. Chicago, IL: Academy of Nutrition and Dietetics; 2013. Reprinted with permission

Physical Activity Coefficients for Healthy-Weight Boys and Girls Ages 3 to 18 Years

| | Physical Activity Coefficient | |
Physical Activity Level[a]	Boys	Girls
Sedentary	1.00	1.00
Low active	1.13	1.16
Active	1.26	1.31
Very active	1.42	1.56

[a] Physical activity level, defined as the ratio of total energy expenditure to basal energy expenditure, is determined by assessing the amount of time the child or adolescent spends in moderate and vigorous play and work.

From Leonberg, BL. *The Academy of Nutrition and Dietetics Pocket Guide to Pediatric Nutrition Assessment*. 2nd ed. Chicago, IL: Academy of Nutrition and Dietetics; 2013. Reprinted with permission.

Appendix B

Examples of Comparative Standards

Estimated Calorie Needs per Day by Age, Sex, and Physical Activity

The Dietary Guidelines assigns individuals to a calorie level based on their sex, age, and activity level. The tables identify the calorie levels for males and females by age and activity level.

See Appendix 2 of the Dietary Guidelines 2005–2020: (https://health.gov/dietaryguidelines/2015/guidelines/appendix-2/).

USDA Food Patterns: Healthy US-Style Eating Pattern: Recommended Amounts of Food From Each Food Group at 12 Calorie Levels

The Dietary Guidelines suggest the amount of food to consume from the basic food groups, subgroups, and oils to meet the recommended intakes at 12 different calorie levels.

See Appendix 3 of the Dietary Guidelines 2005–2020: USDA Food Patterns: Healthy US-Style Eating Pattern: (https://health.gov/dietaryguidelines/2015/guidelines/appendix-3/)

Appendix C

Guidelines for Measuring Height and Weighing Children

How to Measure Weight

Children who are age 2 years or older, cooperative, and able to stand on their own are measured standing.

Equipment

Infants are weighed using an infant pan or table-model scale on a level surface. Children who are able to stand without assistance should be weighed using a platform scale. This may be a beam-balance scale or a digital (electronic load cell or strain gauge) scale. Scales should be calibrated on a routine basis.

Procedure for Weighing Children

1. Remove the child's outer clothing and shoes.
2. Place the scale in the zero position before the child steps on the scale.
3. Have the child stand still with both feet in the center of the platform.
4. Read the measurement to the nearest ¼ pound (100 g) and record results immediately.

How to Measure Height

Children who are age 2 years or older, cooperative, and able to stand on their own are measured standing.

Equipment

A standing height board or stadiometer is required. The device has a flat vertical surface on which a measuring rule is attached. It has a movable headpiece, and either a permanent surface to stand on is provided or the entire device is mounted on the wall of a room with a level floor.

Procedure for Measuring a Child

1. Remove the child's shoed, hat, and bulky clothing, such as coats and sweaters. Undo or adjust hairstyles and remove hair accessories that would interfere with measurement.

2. The child should stand erect, with shoulders level, hands at sides, knees or thighs together, and weight evenly distributed on both feet. The child's feet should be flat on the floor or on a foot piece, with both heels comfortably together and touching the base of the vertical board. When possible, all four contact points (ie, the head, back, buttocks, and heels) should touch the vertical surface while maintaining a natural stance (see Figure C.1). Some children will not be able to maintain a natural stance if all four contact points are touching the vertical surface. For these, at a minimum two contact points—the head and buttocks, or the buttocks and heels—should always touch the vertical surface.

3. Position the child's head by placing a hand on the chin to move the head into the Frankfort plane, as shown in Figure C.1. The Frankfort plane is an imaginary line from the lower margin of the eye socket to the notch above the tragus of the ear. When the child is aligned correctly, the Frankfort plane is parallel to the horizontal headpiece and perpendicular to the vertical back piece of the stadiometer. This is best

    viewed and aligned when the examiner is directly to the side and at eye level with the child.

4. Lower the headpiece until it firmly touches the crown of the head and is at a right angle with the measurement surface. Check contact points as shown in Figure C.1 to ensure that the lower body stays in the proper position and the heels remain flat. Some children may stand up on their toes, but verbal reminders are usually sufficient to get them in the proper position. If a 2-year-old is developmentally immature and cannot follow directions, it may indicate that a recumbent length should be taken instead. Read the stature to the nearest ⅛ inch (1 mm). Record results immediately.

Figure C.1: Positioning a Child Using the Frankfort Plane

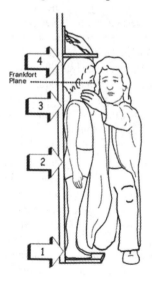

Appendix D

Professional Resources

Centers for Disease Control and Prevention Growth Charts

Downloadable charts are available from the Centers for Disease Control and Prevention (www.cdc.gov/growthcharts). These charts include:

- Weight-for-age percentiles: Boys 2 to 20 years
- Weight-for-age percentiles: Girls 2 to 20 years
- Body mass index (BMI)-for-age percentiles: Boys 2 to 20 years
- BMI-for-age percentiles: Girls 2 to 20 years

The site also includes step-by-step learning modules on BMI, growth charts, and overweight in youth.

Academy of Nutrition and Dietetics

Publications

The following materials and other resources are available at www.eatrightSTORE.org.

- Academy of Nutrition and Dietetics. *Cultural Competency for Nutrition Professionals.* Chicago, IL: Academy of Nutrition and Dietetics; 2015.
- Academy of Nutrition and Dietetics. *Medicare Part B MNT Resources: Become a Provider–Steps to Enroll.* Chicago, IL: Academy of Nutrition and Dietetics; 2011.

- Academy of Nutrition and Dietetics. *Medicare Part B MNT Resources: Overview of the Medicare MNT Benefit.* Chicago, IL: Academy of Nutrition and Dietetics; 2010.
- Academy of Nutrition and Dietetics. *Medicare Part B MNT Resources: A Set of All Handouts.* Chicago, IL: Academy of Nutrition and Dietetics; 2015.
- Academy of Nutrition and Dietetics. *Medicare MNT Provider Newsletter.*
- Behavioral Health Nutrition Dietetic Practice Group and Pediatric Nutrition Practice Group. DeVore J, Shotton A, eds. *Academy of Nutrition and Dietetics Pocket Guide to Children with Special Health Care and Nutritional Needs.* Chicago, IL: Academy of Nutrition and Dietetics; 2012.
- Duyff RL, ed. *Academy of Nutrition and Dietetics Complete Food & Nutrition Guide.* 5th ed. Boston, MA: Houghton Mifflin Harcourt; 2017.
- Kosharek S. *If Your Child Is Overweight: A Guide for Parents.* 4th ed. Chicago, IL: Academy of Nutrition and Dietetics; 2016.
- Leonberg B. *Academy of Nutrition and Dietetics Pocket Guide to Pediatric Nutrition Assessment.* 2nd ed. Chicago, IL: Academy of Nutrition and Dietetics; 2013.
- Pediatric Nutrition Dietetic Practice Group. Groh-Wargo S, Thompson M, Hovasi J, eds. *Academy of Nutrition and Dietetics Pocket Guide to Neonatal Nutrition.* 2nd ed. Chicago, IL: Academy of Nutrition and Dietetics; 2015.
- Pediatric Nutrition Dietetic Practice Group. Kane-Alves V, Tarrant S, eds. *The Nutrition Care Process in Pediatric Practice.* Chicago, IL: Academy of Nutrition and Dietetics; 2013.

- Shield J. Mullen MC. *The Complete Counseling Kit for Pediatric Weight Management.* Chicago, IL: Academy of Nutrition and Dietetics; 2015.
- Shield, J, Mullen MC. *Healthy Eating, Healthy Weight for Kids and Teens.* Chicago, IL: Academy of Nutrition and Dietetics; 2012.
- Silver A, Stollman L. *Making Nutrition Your Business: Building a Successful Private Practice.* 2nd ed. Chicago, IL: Academy of Nutrition and Dietetics; 2017.

Online Resources from the Academy

- Academy of Nutrition and Dietetics. *Nutrition Terminology Reference Manual (eNCPT): Dietetics Language for Nutrition Care, 2014.* Chicago, IL: Academy of Nutrition and Dietetics; 2015. https://ncpt.webauthor.com.
- Academy of Nutrition and Dietetics. *Pediatric Nutrition Care Manual (PNCM).* www.nutritioncaremanual.org.
- Academy of Nutrition and Dietetics. Pediatric Weight Management (PWM) Guideline 2015. www.andeal.org/topic.cfm?menu=5296&cat=5632.
- Academy of Nutrition and Dietetics. Position of the Academy of Nutrition and Dietetics: Interventions for the prevention and treatment of pediatric overweight and obesity. *J Acad Nutr Diet.* 2013;113(10):1375–1394.
- Academy of Nutrition and Dietetics. Position of the Academy of Nutrition and Dietetics: Nutrition guidance for healthy children ages 2 to 11 years. *J Acad Nutr Diet.* 2014;114(8):1257–1276.

Websites

Nutrition and Physical Activity

- Academy of Nutrition and Dietetics. www.eatright.org.
- American Council on Exercise. www.acefitness.org.
- Center for Nutrition Policy and Promotion. www.cnpp.usda.gov.
- Dietary Guidelines for Americans 2015–2020. 8th ed. https://health.gov/dietaryguidelines/.
- Food and Nutrition Information Center. http://fnic.nal.usda.gov.
- Institute of Medicine of the National Academies— Food and Nutrition Topics page. www.iom.edu/Global/Topics/Food-Nutrition.aspx.
- International Food Information Council Foundation. http://ific.org.
- Kids Eat Right. www.kidseatright.org.
- Let's Move. www.letsmove.gov.
- Maternal and Child Health Library. www.ncemch.org/mchlibrary.ph.
- National Association for Health and Fitness. www.physicalfitness.org.
- National Recreation and Park Association. www.nrpa.org.
- Nutrition.gov (gateway to US government nutrition information). www.nutrition.gov.
- President's Council on Physical Fitness and Sports. www.fitness.gov.
- Society of Health and Physical Educators (SHAPE America). www.shapeamerica.org.
- US Department of Agriculture Cooperative State Research, Education, and Extension Service. https://nifa.usda.gov.

- US Department of Agriculture My Plate. www.choosemyplate.gov.

Health and Disease Prevention/Treatment

- American Academy of Family Physicians. www.aafp.org.
- American Academy of Pediatrics. www.aap.org.
- American Cancer Society. www.cancer.org.
- American Diabetes Association. www.diabetes.org.
- American Heart Association. www.heart.org.
- American Medical Association. www.ama-assn.org.
- American Nurses Association. www.ana.org.
- American Psychological Association. www.apa.org.
- American Public Health Association. www.apha.org.
- Bright Futures at Georgetown University. www.brightfutures.org.
- Centers for Disease Control and Prevention. www.cdc.gov.
- Food and Drug Administration. www.fda.gov.
- Office of Disease Prevention and Health Promotion: Healthfinder. http://healthfinder.gov.
- Maternal and Child Health Bureau. http://mchb.hrsa.gov.
- National Association of Pediatric Nurse Practitioners. www.napnap.org.
- National Association of Social Workers. www.socialworkers.org.
- National Cancer Institute. www.cancer.gov.
- National Center for Education in Maternal and Child Health. www.ncemch.org.
- National Center for Health Statistics. www.cdc.gov/nchs.
- National Heart, Lung, and Blood Institute. www.nhlbi.nih.gov.

- National Institute of Child Health and Human Development. www.nichd.nih.gov.
- National Institute of Diabetes and Digestive and Kidney Disease. www.niddk.nih.gov.
- National Institutes of Health. http://health.nih.gov.
- Office of Disease Prevention and Health Promotion. http://health.gov.
- US Department of Health and Human Services. www.hhs.gov.

Eating Disorders and Body Image

- Academy for Eating Disorders. www.aedweb.org.
- GirlsHealth.gov. www.girlshealth.gov/
- National Association of Anorexia Nervosa and Associated Disorders. www.anad.org.
- National Eating Disorders Association. www.nationaleatingdisorders.org.
- National Women's Health Information Center. www.womenshealth.gov.

Healthy Weight and Overweight

- Academy of Nutrition and Dietetics. www.eatright.org.
- American Heart Association: Childhood Obesity. www.heart.org/HEARTORG /GettingHealthy /HealthierKids/ChildhoodObesity/What-is-childhood-obesity_UCM_304347_Article.jsp.
- Healthy Weight Network. www.healthyweight.net.
- National Heart, Lung, and Blood Institute, Obesity Education Initiative. www.nhlbi.nih.gov/about/oei/index.htm.
- The Obesity Society. www.obesity.org.

- We Can! (Ways to Enhance Children's Activity and Nutrition). www.nhlbi.nih.gov/health/public/heart /obesity/wecan.
- Weight-Control Information Center. http://win.niddk.nih.gov/index.htm.

Other Online Resources

- The National Diabetes Education Program of the Centers for Disease Control and Prevention offers a variety of resources relevant to Asian American, Native Hawaiian, and Pacific Islander populations with or at risk for diabetes, including many in a variety of non-English languages. www.cdc.gov/diabetes/ndep/resources-for-aa-nh-pi.htm.
- FDA Office of Women's Health offers free health publications in multiple foreign languages, including some on heart health and osteoporosis. www.fda.gov/For Consumers/ByAudience/ForWomen/FreePublications /ucm116738.htm.
- US Department of Agriculture Food and Nutrition Information Center, Ethnic and Cultural Resources. http://fnic.nal.usda.gov/professional-and-career-resources/ethnic-and-cultural-resources.
- US Department of Health and Human Services, Outreach Activities & Resources Specialized Information Services. Multi-Cultural Resources for Health Information. http://sis.nlm.nih.gov/outreach/multicultural.html.

Continuing Professional Education

This edition of the *Academy of Nutrition and Dietetics Pocket Guide to Pediatric Weight Management*, Second Edition, offers readers 6 hours of Continuing Professional Education (CPE) credit.

Readers may earn credit by completing the interactive online quiz at: https://publications.webauthor.com/pg _to_pediatric_weight_management_2e.

Index

Page number followed by *b* indicates box; *f*, figure; *t*, table.

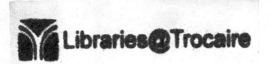